ALL YOUR FAVORITE DISHES!

The average American eats out four times a week! That gets expensive. Now Todd Wilbur shows you how to duplicate at home the taste of the menu items you love—and save a lot of money.

SHONEY'S® HOT FUDGE CAKE
Menu cost: $1.89 Home Version: $0.65

How do you make it? You buy a prepackaged devil's food cake mix, a half-gallon container of vanilla ice cream, a jar of chocolate fudge topping, a can of whipped cream, 12 maraschino cherries— and follow Todd Wilbur's foolproof step-by-step instructions. And if you can't eat it all—he tells you how to freeze it too.

**Over 100 favorite dishes from
Bennigan's®, Big Boy®, The Cheesecake Factory®,
Chili's® Grill and Bar, Hard Rock® Cafe,
Lone Star Steakhouse & Saloon®, Outback Steakhouse®,
Planet Hollywood®, Ruby Tuesday®,
Tony Roma's A Place for Ribs® . . . and more!**

TODD WILBUR is the bestselling author of *Top Secret Recipes* and *More Top Secret Recipes* (both Plume). When not taste-testing recipes on himself, his friends, or TV talk-show hosts, he lives in Las Vegas, Nevada.

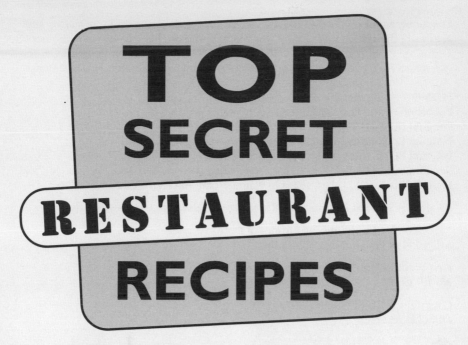

TOP SECRET RESTAURANT RECIPES

Creating Kitchen Clones from America's Favorite Restaurant Chains

✳ ✳ ✳

Todd Wilbur

with Illustrations by the Author

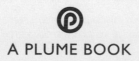

A PLUME BOOK

This book is not authorized by, and neither the author nor the publisher is affiliated with, the restaurants or the owners of the trademarks referred to in the book. Terms mentioned in this book that are known or believed to be trademarks or service marks have been indicated as such in the section "Trademarks" (see Contents).

PLUME
Published by the Penguin Group
Penguin Books USA Inc., 375 Hudson Street, New York, New York 10014, U.S.A.
Penguin Books Ltd, 27 Wrights Lane, London W8 5TZ, England
Penguin Books Australia Ltd, Ringwood, Victoria, Australia
Penguin Books Canada Ltd, 10 Alcorn Avenue, Toronto, Ontario, Canada M4V 3B2
Penguin Books (N.Z.) Ltd, 182–190 Wairau Road, Auckland 10, New Zealand

Penguin Books Ltd, Registered Offices: Harmondsworth, Middlesex, England

First published by Plume, an imprint of Dutton Signet,
a division of Penguin Books USA Inc.

First Printing, June 1997
20 19 18 17

Ⓟ REGISTERED TRADEMARK—MARCA REGISTRADA

LIBRARY OF CONGRESS CATALOGING-IN-PUBLICATION DATA
Wilbur, Todd.
  Top secret restaurant recipes : creating kitchen clones from America's favorite restaurant chains / Todd Wilbur : with illustrations by the author.
    p.   cm.
  ISBN 0-452-27587-3
  1. Cookery, American.   2. Chain restaurants—United States.
I. Title.
TX715.W6587   1997   96-49396
641.5973—dc21   CIP

Printed in the United States of America
Set in Garamond Light and Opti-Adrift
Designed by Eve L. Kirch

BOOKS ARE AVAILABLE AT QUANTITY DISCOUNTS WHEN USED TO PROMOTE PRODUCTS OR SERVICES. FOR INFORMATION PLEASE WRITE TO PREMIUM MARKETING DIVISION, PENGUIN BOOKS USA INC., 375 HUDSON STREET, NEW YORK, NEW YORK 10014.

To the glittering city of Las Vegas,
my new home and a mecca for restaurant chains.
Unfortunately, it also happens to be
the gambling capital of the world, so dining out ends up
costing five times what it used to.

THANK YOU ...

* * *

Arnold Dolin, Lori Lipsky, Alicia Brooks, Ellen Geiger, Tracey Guest, Eve Kirch, Rena Kornbluh, Cheryl Hoffman, Melissa Jacoby, Donna Linderman, Carole DeSanti, Julia Moskin, Amy Mintzer, Plume, Mom, Dad, Scott, Granny, Zebu the Wonder Dog, Scott and Sandy Layer, Dennis Palumbo, Big Al, Dr. Scott Smith & Shannon & Little Al, Felipe Bascope, Tom Ardizzone, Andy & Lorrie, Howard Stern, Maury Povich, *Talk Soup*, Mike & Maty, Pat Bullard, *Crook & Chase*, Christina Ferrare, Chuck Woolery, *HomeMatters*, Jm J. Bullock, Tammy Faye, Ronnie Rubino, LightWave 3D, Cafe Lattes, A Positive Count, General Electric Kitchen VCR/TV, Discovery Channel, Comedy Channel, HBO, Amigas & Pentiums, Chapstick, Basil, Parsley, Cilantro, Thyme, Habañeros, Rapid-O-Graph, *The Larry Sanders Show*, Sarah, Bush, Natalie, Cult, X, Lenny, Alice, S.T.P., Kurt, Hard Rock Hotel, Lounge Chairs, Summerlin, Coyote Cafe, Oscar, Jacuzzis, Fresh Powder, and Beer.

CONTENTS

✳ ✳ ✳

INTRODUCTION

✳ ✳ ✳

N ow it's time for something a little different.

It was a blast writing the first two *Top Secret Recipes* cookbooks that include secret recipes inspired by convenience food—both fast food and packaged food, like Big Macs, Snickers, Oreos, and Twinkies. Sure, dissecting hamburgers, candy bars, cookies, and snack cakes is strange, sticky, tedious work; but when long-time aficionados of these goodies claim the copycat recipe was "right on," or when a blindfolded talk-show host is genuinely fooled in a taste test on live TV, I have to feel encouraged to continue the quest for clones.

So, as I was mulling over the next Top Secret mission, I noticed that in 1996 America would reach a milestone in the full-service restaurant business. For the first time ever in one year, our hungry nation would spend a gastronomic $100 billion, gobbling up the sit-down meals prepared by these rapidly expanding chains— casual diners and steakhouses like Big Boy, The Olive Garden, Outback, Chili's, and Applebee's. That got me thinking. In light of this landmark occasion, it seemed the perfect time for *Top Secret Recipes* to shift its focus, do a little snooping around in the full-service sector, and clone some dishes from the popular restaurant chains Americans have been frequenting in record numbers. But,

1

wait a minute—we're not just talking about cookies and burgers here. These are sit-down meals, with appetizers, entrees, side dishes, and desserts . . . from chains all over the country. Would this be an impossible mission? Eagerly I chose to accept it. And I'm happy to say after more than a year of tasty field work: mission accomplished!

The Criteria

The casual and fine dining restaurant chains that are referred to as "full-service" in the food biz are the sole subject of this formula-cracking volume. Just for clarity's sake, "full-service" excludes "quick-service" or "fast food" restaurants. That means you won't find recipes here for Wendy's or Taco Bell or Burger King where you order your paper-wrapped food over a counter or from a drive-thru window (look for those recipes in the previous two *Top Secret Recipes* volumes).

At a full-service chain you typically order from a menu while sitting down at a private table. You are usually waited on, you can order a beer, you can pay with a credit card, and you are expected to leave a tip. A full-service restaurant can be a steakhouse, a family diner, a casual dinner house, a fancy restaurant, or extravagant theme chain.

Altogether, the selection of restaurants represented here total 19,000 single outlets grossing more than $25 billion a year. Many of the chains are at the top of the list in annual sales figures, but to maintain a bit of variety, I've picked some chains that are smaller in total size with only a regional presence. A few of the chains represented are located mostly in the South, such as Cracker Barrel, Western Sizzlin', and Shoney's; some are more likely to be found in the Northeast, such as Chi-Chi's and Perkins; and a couple of the chains come from the West, like Marie Callender's and Stuart Anderson's Black Angus. You'll also find that many of the chains are national, like the ubiquitous Pizza Hut, Red Lobster, and Denny's. A book like this wouldn't be complete without recognizing the ultra-hot theme restaurant segment, which includes Hard Rock Cafe, Planet Hollywood, and Dive!.

2

TOP 10 FULL-SERVICE RESTAURANT CHAINS

Rank	Restaurant	'95 U.S. Units	'95 Sales ($MM)
1.	Pizza Hut	12,140	7,900.0
2.	Red Lobster	727	1,930.0
3.	Denny's	1,553	1,490.0
4.	Shoney's	822	1,260.4
5.	The Olive Garden	494	1,260.0
6.	Applebee's	666	1,250.0
7.	Chili's Grill & Bar	490	1,060.0
8.	T.G.I. Friday's	535	1,043.0
9.	Big Boy	850	970.0
10.	Outback Steakhouse	320	827.0

Source: Restaurants & Institutions

Because the average American eats out 198 times a year or 4 times a week, chances are very good that you've noshed at one or more of these establishments in the past. You may even be familiar with several of the dishes that inspired the recipes in this book. That's good. Now you can take the *Top Secret Recipes* taste test. Compare what you make to the original menu item and you should find your version tastes just like the dish from the restaurant. To ensure that this is the case, I've tested the recipes numerous times. If my version didn't taste like the real dish, it didn't go in the book. Sure, the *Top Secret Recipes* version may not be prepared the exact same way as the original, but as long as the finished product is identical in taste, how we get to that point is inconsequential. Be aware that my intention here is not to steal the original recipe from the creators, only to duplicate the finished product as closely as possible, with ingredients you can find in any supermarket.

I've had to visit most of these restaurants several times to obtain all of the necessary information to assemble the recipes. Any information I obtained about these dishes came from talking to servers or hosts/hostesses (some more cooperative than others), just as any other customer might ask about a particular dish. Everything else I needed to know came from examining the dish itself.

You'd think that I was the only goofball out there traveling from

3

restaurant to restaurant, quizzing waitresses and cooks, loading leftovers into Tupperware and Ziploc bags under dining room tables and into coolers stashed in car trunks. But there are many other more professional and much sneakier sleuths out there working for major restaurant companies, whose job it is to analyze the competitors' high-profit dishes and create a version for their own chain. If they succeed, they'll put those dishes on their own menu, maybe change the dish just slightly, and give it a new name.

You may not know that the double decker Big Mac, which I cloned in a previous book, is not McDonald's own creation as many would believe, but rather a knock-off of the double-decker sandwich first created by the founder of the Big Boy chain 30 years before it was served under the Golden Arches (Big Boy's version is included in this book). On many menus today you'll find a common appetizer called potato skins, but you probably didn't know that it was T.G.I. Friday's that first introduced the dish to the world in 1974. And more recently, the popular fried Bloomin' Onion that was created by one of the Outback Steakhouse founders has become one of the most duplicated appetizers today, complete with the spicy dipping sauce and different names like "Awesome Blossom" and "Texas Tumbleweed."

Why Clone?

In the competitive arena of food service where the failure rate is a brutal 85 percent, operators are masters at inventing new and exciting dishes, creating new trends, or further exploiting existing ones and building menus around them . . . even if a bit of cloning goes on. Successful restaurant operators are adept at attacking our taste buds with a flavorful frontal assault that will make us come back for more.

The recipes picked for this book should tickle your taste buds the same way as their original counterparts. Sure, making these dishes at home is not as easy as going out to the restaurant, and there's no way this book can substitute for the experience of dining out and mingling with others in a relaxing environment. That's why a book like this could never put a dent in the profit margin of these large chains. But when the time comes that you decide you want to do some cooking of your own, perhaps some entertaining, now you've got some tasty and familiar alternatives for the menu. Beyond that, I think you'll find home-cloning has additional benefits:

Because several of the restaurants are regional, there's no place in the entire country where you can get everything represented here. Making the dish at home is one way to find out how the other half dines. If you live on the West Coast you can enjoy East Coast fare like the food from Chi-Chi's or Cracker Barrel without having to take a very, very long drive. That is, until these chains expand into your neck of the woods.

Secondly, dining out regularly can get to be quite expensive. Sure, you don't want to have to cook all of the time, but why not stay in and make your favorite restaurant dishes at home once in a while to save a little cash? From this purely random selection you can see the big savings:

Planet Hollywood Chicken Crunch	Menu: $6.50	Home version: $2.12
Applebee's Quesadillas	Menu: $4.99	Home version: $1.11
Shoney's Hot Fudge Cake	Menu: $1.89	Home version: $0.65

Restaurants have to price their products to pay for operating overhead like servers, managers and chefs, leases and advertising. Your dish will cost less since you don't have these sorts of expenses.

Thirdly, you can alter the dishes to suit your taste. If you need your version of the Bloomin' Onion dipping sauce a little spicier, add more horseradish or cayenne pepper. If you want the sauce to be lower in calories, use a light mayonnaise that can be found in practically every market these days. Experiment and customize the dishes to suit your dietary needs and preferences.

You also have the ability now to create menus for entire meals that consist of a mix of dishes from different restaurants. You might try the clone recipe for Outback's Walkabout Soup as an appetizer, followed by the Western T-bone from Stuart Anderson's

Black Angus, with a side of Texas Rice from Lone Star. Follow that up with a Strawberry Tallcake for Two from Ruby Tuesday and you've just eaten a meal that you could only get from lots of traveling around with doggie bags.

Here are some other suggestions:

For dinner:
> Shoney's Slow-Cooked Pot Roast
> Houlihan's Smashed Potatoes
> Sizzler Cheese Toast
> Cheesecake Factory Key Lime Cheesecake

Or:
> Houlihan's Houli Fruit Fizz
> T.G.I. Friday's Potato Skins
> Tony Roma's Original Baby Back Ribs
> Bennigan's Cookie Mountain Sundae

Or:
> Hooters Buffalo Shrimp
> California Pizza Kitchen Thai Chicken Pizza
> Chi-Chi's Mexican "Fried" Ice Cream

For an old-fashioned, country-style dinner:
> Marie Callender's Famous Golden Cornbread
> Shoney's Country Fried Steak
> Houlihan's Smashed Potatoes
> Marie Callender's Banana Cream Pie

For an Italian dinner:
> Cheesecake Factory Bruschetta
> Olive Garden Toscana Soup
> Planet Hollywood Pizza Bread
> Olive Garden Alfredo Pasta

For a little surf and turf:
> Salad w/Olive Garden Italian Salad Dressing
> Stuart Anderson's Black Angus Cheesy Garlic Bread

Red Lobster Broiled Lobster
Ruth's Chris Petite Filet
Ruth's Chris Creamed Spinach or Potatoes Au Gratin

For breakfast:
Cracker Barrel Hash Brown Casserole
Perkins Country Club Omelette

For lunch:
Hooters Pasta Salad
Dive! Sicilian Sub Rosa
Hard Rock Cafe Orange Freeze

For the vegetarian:
Dive! Carrot Chips
Big Boy Cream of Broccoli Soup
Hard Rock Cafe Grilled Vegetable Sandwich
Shoney's Hot Fudge Cake

For munching while watching the big game:
Hooters Buffalo Chicken Wings
Olive Garden Hot Artichoke & Spinach Dip
Pizza Hut Original Stuffed Crust Pizza

For a party:
T.G.I. Friday's Nine-Layer Dip
Applebee's Pizza Sticks
Outback Gold Coast Coconut Shrimp
Hard Rock Cafe Watermelon Ribs
Ruth's Chris Potatoes Au Gratin
Red Robin Mountain High Mudd Pie
T.G.I. Friday's Smoothies

These are just some ideas. Surely there are many great combinations of these dishes, and I'm sure you can come up with some of your own that will include clones of creations from the restaurants that you like best.

Lastly, just for fun, you'd like to know if this smarty-pants author can really do what he says he can—create recipes that taste just like the real deal. Take the Top Secret Challenge. Get some of these dishes to go, make the clone, put on some blindfolds and give it the true taste test. If all goes well, you should have a tough time identifying the real product over the phony. My fingers are crossed.

Some Quick Tips

To help ensure that all goes well, here are some quick words of advice on how to use this book to get the best results from your cloning experience:

- Read the entire recipe through before you start cooking. There's been many a time I didn't familiarize myself with a recipe first, only to discover halfway through that I wouldn't be able to finish, since I didn't have the right equipment or ingredients. You will need to know if you'll be using the barbecue, so you can refill the propane that ran out last Saturday. You will want to know that you need an 8-inch springform pan before you start the cheesecake. Read ahead and minimize the surprises.
- Read the "Tidbits" section at the end of any recipe that has one. That section may offer some helpful advice or recipe variations you might want to try.
- Know the yield before you start. I've designed several of the recipes, especially sandwiches, to yield only enough for one serving, but those recipes can be easily doubled, tripled, or quadrupled to serve more.
- Refer to the "blueprints." Each of the recipes has been written so that you shouldn't need to refer to a drawing for help. But, you'll find the drawings give you a good idea what you're shooting for. As they say, a picture is worth a thousand words. When it comes to kitchen cloning, perhaps it's worth even more than that.
- Identify parts of the recipes that can be used for other dishes. Many of the recipes include dips, dressings, and sauces which are great stand-alone recipes to use in another dish you may

8

create. You may find that the teriyaki sauce in the Western Sizzlin' "Teriyaki" Chicken or the honey-lime dressing for Chili's Caribbean Chicken Salad can be used as delicious marinades in other recipes.

So, clone away and, most important, have fun with it. I hope you enjoy trying these recipes as much as I did creating them. Perhaps many will become permanent additions to your home menus.

I'd love to hear if you have any requests for additional recipes in future volumes of *Top Secret Recipes* as many of the recipes in this book started with a request from readers like you. If you have a favorite product or dish you'd like to see cloned you can send your suggestions to me at:

Todd Wilbur—Top Secret Recipes
c/o Penguin USA
375 Hudson Street
New York, NY 10014–3657

I promise to read your letter as soon as I get the hardened dough out from under my fingernails.

TABLE FOR TWO:
THE RESTAURANT TALE

✳ ✳ ✳

Somewhere around 1500 B.C. in ancient Egypt, the first full-service food establishment on the planet opened its doors. No one is sure of the name; so we'll just call it "Happy Joseph's Nile Inn." You see, Joe, the proprietor, was a bright man. His ancestors had been prospering for thousands of years, with everything they required to lead comfortable lives being provided by the rich, fertile lands surrounding the nearby Nile River. But, you know how it is—give an ancient Egyptian a millennium or two, and he's going to want more than the same old figs and geese and robes and jewelry enjoyed by his great-great-great-great-great-great-great grandparents.

Happy Joe was a thoughtful man who watched as merchants set out in large caravans on journeys to great lands hundreds of miles away. The melange of cloth, tools, fruits, vegetables, and livestock that these merchants brought back would make them wealthy and popular. Soon many more merchants seeking similar wealth would set out on such journeys in search of better weapons, more colorful dyes, and a beer that still tasted great, but was a little less filling.

Joe knew these weary travelers would require a cozy place to stop, kick off the sandals, and get some shuteye for the night; a place that could shelter them from the cold and offer them some nourishment. The trips were treacherous, filled with adventure, and plagued by robbers—this was work that made a man ravenous and weary. Happy Joseph's Nile Inn provided the men with a welcome bellyful of grub and a cozy bed of straw in exchange for precious goods off their wagons.

Though this may have been the first restaurant in the world, it bore little similarity to the restaurants we know today. When you stopped in at Happy Joe's you wouldn't have been seated at a private table by a smiling hostess, nor would you choose your meal from a colorful menu, nor would you eat your food with a fork or knife. At Joe's place there was one long wooden table where everybody sat to eat and you picked your entree from the livestock or produce you carried with you on your journey (yes, it was B.Y.O.). Joe merely prepared it for you using his own knives and pots and a great little charcoal stove that worked much like the stoves we use today. Joe grilled your antelope meat and offered you beer or wine, while his wife baked delicious bread. When the food was ready you helped yourself and sat on a bench to eat with your fingers. Then you cheerfully passed out in the corner amongst a pile of your companions.

Happy Joe's became exceedingly popular. But time eventually took its toll and Joe grew too old for the work. One day he and his wife closed up the business for good and retired to a small southern beach community.

Though he did marvelous things with gazelle butt steaks, Joe's food would hardly be missed. By then many other entrepreneurs had followed in Joe's footsteps to open their own inns along the expanding trade routes. Eventually this included the entire eastern end of the Mediterranean Sea. By now these inns were providing their own food—no longer did you have to bring it with you. If you arrived at the right time, you could help yourself to a share of whatever was cooking in the pot or baking in the stove. If you got there late in the evening, you had better like your meat very well done, cold, or both. That is, if there was any left.

These inns were soon offering more comforts and pleasures to the weary travelers. Prostitution became a popular service exchanged for money and goods in these establishments. Merchants served coffees and pastries to the customers—predecessors to today's popular coffeehouses (which generally lack the carnal offerings). The menus were improving considerably at these inns, which were now selling a variety of foods including fresh vegetables and fruits, fish, duck, goose, beef, milk, cheese, butter, fancy cakes, date and palm wine, and beer. This was a time of great growth and development in the early food-service business, for many of the same techniques of food preparation that we use today have origins in ancient Egypt. Nevertheless, historians still argue amongst themselves whether this is when the slogan "Eat at Joe's" was first used.

Grease in Greece

In 1000 B.C. the center of civilization moved up the eastern end of the Mediterranean and then west to Greece. Here, it was the duty of the slaves to do all of the cooking. At first, the slaves were female—just about every household had a couple—with very basic cooking skills. Then there began a shift toward male slaves who were very skilled in all aspects of cooking. These special slaves, or *magieros,* gained much respect for their duties in the kitchen. A magiero was encouraged to develop new dishes and earned public acclaim for fancy feasts prepared by assistants under his control. These were the original chefs responsible for making the art of cooking a respectable profession.

Those ancient Greeks, what trendsetters they were. It was the Greeks who developed the custom of three meals that is familiar in much of the world today, although the types of food eaten at these meals has changed significantly. For example, shortly after getting out of bed it was customary to eat a meal called *ariston,* which included bread dipped in wine. Just try explaining that one at work. The next meal was called *diepnon* and was eaten shortly after noon. It consisted of a dish that varied from household to household, but could have included breads, cakes and porridge, vegetables and fruits, plus eggs, poultry, or fish. The main meal of the day would come shortly after sunset and was called *cena* or *derpon.* This meal, like our dinner, consisted of meat with vegetables and bread or other side dishes, and a dessert. The Greeks used olive oil in place of butter and they sweetened their food with honey.

The ancient Greeks loved to eat in groups. They would throw huge parties in dining clubs and gorge themselves with food prepared by magieros and their apprentices. This was their version of the full-service restaurant. The custom was to lie on the left side on rows of cushioned couches and eat with the right hand from baskets of food brought to them. There were no utensils to speak of except maybe a spoonlike implement used to handle gravies, sauces, and soups. The only knife in the dining room was handled by the carver, whose job it was to ensure that everyone's meat had been cut into bite-size pieces. "Oh, carve boy! Chop-chop."

In 146 B.C. the Romans conquered the Greeks, and that was the end of that party.

When in Rome

Although handy in a battle, the ancient Romans were pigs. On a daily basis they would eat all their meals at one sitting that would start at around one o'clock in the afternoon, after the close of business. Then they would eat and eat and eat, sometimes through the night and into the next day. The Roman emperor Nero had been known to eat continuously for thirty-six hours.

The first part of the meal was *gustaus,* which might include eggs, vegetables, and shellfish. The main course, or *mensa prima,* consisted of stews or roasted veal, fish, or fowl. For dessert, *mensa secunda,* came pastries, honey-sweetened cakes, fruits, jams, and sweetmeats. On special occasions this afternoon meal was expanded to include six courses or more. But that was nothing. It was in the commonly celebrated banquets and dinner parties that Romans demonstrated their hedonistic and gastronomic overindulgences.

You'd be challenged to find an establishment that throws a party like those the Romans enjoyed. Huge sums of money were spent and crowds of people would jam into extravagantly furnished dining halls. Sandals were removed and feet were washed by slaves. Upon cloth-covered tables was served course after course of food and wine. Guests used spoons and forks and knives and toothpicks to eat from ornate serving platters. They were required to bring their own napkins, but that was okay, since they could wrap up leftovers to take home—the first doggie bags!

Several hours into these dinner parties, when the guests could eat no more, they would force themselves to vomit, and start all over again. As this went on for seven, eight, nine hours, and as the wine was taking its toll, robes were removed and the party degenerated into a huge sexual orgy. The slaves that earlier had been serving food would now be beaten for amusement and the banquet hall would be in shambles.

Sure, this sounds more like a college frat party than a dining experience, but the Romans also had establishments that somewhat resembled our modern restaurants. They were called *taberna meritoria* or taverns of merit. Here guests would sit in dining halls at long tables and were served food while the proprietor watched from a raised platform at the front of the room. If the food was not satisfactory the cook would be flogged in the dining room. This little incentive encouraged a culinary artistry similar to that of the ancient Greeks, with care taken to present the food most elegantly.

Magieros continued to teach the Romans about cooking and many were freed by grateful masters who appreciated their skill in the kitchen. The kitchen was now separated from other rooms and departmentalized, and the first cookbook was written during this era, by Apicus, in A.D. 25. The title, crudely translated: "Please Don't Flog Before You Try My Grilled Hog."

The Middle Ages Sucked

The Middle or Dark Ages added virtually nothing to our cuisine or dining customs. When the Greek and Roman empires vanished, records of their culinary achievements were left undiscovered until after the demise of this medieval era.

For the next 1400 years, civilization in Europe seemed to move backward into a dark time where kings ruled from cold stone castles and the lower classes lived in small mud or thatch huts. While poor farmers were living on tiny meals of turnips, cabbage, and salt pork, feudal rulers were stuffing themselves on as many as thirty meals a day. Still, the food was bland and stuck together with thick sauces and gravies so that it could be eaten with only the hands. Utensils and plates were not used. The food was cut into bite-size portions and poured into hollowed-out loaves of bread called "trenchers." A spoonlike implement had been developed, but it was so difficult to use, everyone preferred to use their fingers.

In the castles, meals were served in huge dining halls filled with hundreds of people who just stood around talking until they could take their turn at the grub. The room was usually filled with smoke from a huge fire blazing in the center of the room. Knights would bring their horses into the hall, so that they would be ready for battle, and dogs were rummaging through the straw for bones and scraps of food. This loud, smelly occasion was more like a dirt-cheap, Podunk wedding reception from hell, than a time to enjoy a decent meal. Let's set that clock forward, quick.

Now We're Getting There

The 1500s saw a noticeable improvement in food and culinary artistry, at last. Spices were coming in from the Orient to put some zing into the bland, nearly tasteless food of the Middle Ages. The kingdoms were dissolving and people were beginning to rediscover food.

In the seventeenth century, the table fork was reintroduced to the world. This was significant for the changes the implement would bring to the consistency and form of food. The sticky goo that had become an important ingredient in finger food of the Dark Ages was no longer a necessity. Shortly thereafter the dinner plate that had been missing from food service since Roman times was back, and the culinary arts flourished.

Chefs designed creative and tasty dishes, and brought a new era of professionalism to the industry. The highly talented chefs gained a great deal of respect and wealth, and dressed as noblemen.

The eighteenth century saw rapid growth throughout Europe. Because of this, meat, bread, and other foods were in scarce supply. So the King of France established a system that gave exclusive rights to a group of cooks to sell specific prepared meals. This small group of cooks offered these high-quality, expensive meals to only those who could afford them. Other, less wealthy customers had to settle for the lower-quality, meatless food prepared by soup vendors.

One of these merchants was Boulanger, a man who, in 1765, saw a need for more substance in his dishes. He had no license to sell meat, but had created a soup consisting of sheep's feet in cream sauce (Mmm, mmm good). To sell his soup he couldn't mention meat, or risk arrest, so he put a sign over his shop which said, "Boulanger sells magical restoratives." The dish was a big hit and his shop became very popular. Soon the word "restorative" evolved into "restaurant," now the accepted term for an establishment committed solely to the business of providing meals to the public.

It didn't take long for restaurants to start popping up all over the place throughout France. The French Revolution forced many of the wealthy aristocrats to lose valuable property, so they had to let go of their private chefs. With nothing else to do, these talented artisans opened their own restaurants, and soon there was a surge of fancy eateries. By 1804, Paris boasted more than 400 restaurants, many of them responsible for creating scores of now-famous dishes—a redeeming factor for a nation that 150 years later would consider Jerry Lewis a genius.

First on the Block in America

In Boston, a man named Samuel Cole saw the opportunity to pocket some serious coin from the increasing number of travelers along a major roadway, much like his Egyptian predecessor, Happy Joe. So, in 1734, he opened up a joint called "Cole's" to service the constant flow of stagecoaches full of hungry travelers. Sammy referred to his new place as an "ordinary," or "tavern," which was just another name for an "inn" in New England. But, unlike everyone else in the inn business, Sammy didn't take overnight guests (and he didn't take American Express). This set Cole's apart from the rest as the first establishment to concentrate on preparing and serving food to guests who would not be spending the night. Cole's became America's first restaurant.

Through the 1700s, taverns dotted the roadsides as settlers migrated across America. The food served in these establishments remained unexciting, ordinary fare, served from a kettle which hung over a flame in the fireplace. But in 1827, that would begin to change. This was the year that John Delmonico, a Swiss immigrant, opened the world-renowned restaurant Delmonico's in New York City.

Delmonico's brought a touch of class to the food-service industry.

17

The restaurant served food with great attention to every aspect of its preparation and presentation. Its extensive menu was printed in both French and English, and every waiter was bilingual. At Delmonico's you dined at cloth-covered tables, you chose your wine from an extensive list, and enjoyed a wide selection of European entrees never before served in the United States. All of this while surrounded by a clientele from the upper crust, including businessmen and statesmen, presidents and dignitaries.

Delmonico's attention to detail set the pace for fancy restaurants that would come in future years, many of them directly influenced by John Delmonico's concept. Delmonico would even copy himself, by opening up branches of his own restaurant in other locations—a trend very popular today. Delmonico's was the first documented restaurant in the U.S. to serve "Hamburg Steak," a broiled chopped steak dish that would evolve into America's most popular food: the hamburger.

The original Delmonico's survived for 96 years, finally closing its doors in 1923, but not before making the full-service fine dining experience a popular institution.

Modern Developments at Last

As the world's first cafeteria was being created in San Francisco during the gold rush of 1849, significant developments were being made in kitchen equipment. In 1850 the cast iron stove was invented. It gave way to the gas stove in the 1870s as lines were built to pump gas into the growing cities. By 1889, the hot water heater was created, which helped dishwashers to clean dishes without tying up the stove with pots of boiling water. Food that had been stored in simple iceboxes (metal boxes with ice in them) was now being stored in mechanical, ammonia-driven refrigerators. These creations would help to improve the quality of food served in restaurants into the twentieth century and beyond.

As the 1900s rolled around, several new inventions were being put to the test in the company restaurant at the Sears and Roebuck mail-order firm in Chicago. The company had just opened the largest food-service operation in the world to feed its employees at lunchtime. And, oh, what a lunchtime it was! One hundred employees operated five restaurants with two thousand seats; they served 12,500 meals a day. A machine made ice around the clock and dishes were washed by an automatic dishwashing machine. Automation was leading to more efficiency in the kitchen, so that restaurants could serve customers faster, and be prepared for the next arrivals instantaneously.

Food service was getting better and faster. With the popularity of cars on the rise, Roy Allen devised the first drive-in refreshment stand with carhop service in Lodi, California. When Allen later teamed up with Frank Wright, signs would be raised with the initials "A&W," marking a growing number of root beer outlets that all became part of the world's first franchise.

Two years later Royce Hailey would open the first of many Pig Stands in Dallas, Texas, serving sandwiches hot off the grill to customers who drove up in their cars. By 1930 there were thirty Pig Stands across the country, and carhop service evolved into a drive-up window, much like those we're used to today. Fast food had arrived.

Table for Two

When alcohol was put on a nationwide ban in 1919, soda fountains got a boost in popularity as people looked for a refreshing recreational replacement. Prior to prohibition the pharmacist would be the one to supply the alcohol, so naturally the drugstores became host to the many soda fountains, serving ice cream, root beer, and tonics. Pharmacists were eager to replace their lost alcohol sales.

One day while working as a concessionaire at a soda fountain in the Franklin Institute exhibit in Philadelphia, Robert Green ran out of the cream that was used in one of the popular refreshments. He substituted a large scoop of ice cream and at that moment created the first ice-cream soda. He liked what he tasted and immediately added the cool beverage to the menu. By the end of the exhibition, word had spread of the ice-cream soda and the excitement put about $600 a day into Robert's pocket.

As word got out about this new creation, the phenomenon of the ice-cream soda soon spread across the country. Fountains were serving the drink regularly to customers, and in consequence more fountains were opening in drugstores, in markets, and on street corners.

One of the drugstores that had been losing money was purchased in 1925 by a guy named Howard Johnson. He served his homemade ice cream and ice-cream sodas at the soda fountain inside the drugstore, but soon added hot dogs and hamburgers to the menu. When he began to turn a profit, Howard turned the drugstore into a restaurant and expanded into other regions. Howard Johnson became the first person to establish a mass-market menu for a full-service restaurant chain.

In 1936, Bob Wian was set on buying a ten-stool hamburger stand in Glendale, California, from a couple of elderly ladies. Since he couldn't pony up the cash, he sold his prized 1933 DeSoto roadster for $350 and secured the deal. He called his new restaurant "Bob's Pantry," a name that would only last a short while.

When Bob created his now-famous double-decker hamburger dubbed "the Big Boy," Bob quickly changed the name of his restaurant chain and franchised like crazy. Big Boy restaurants dotted the nation, and by the time he was thinking about retirement in 1960, Bob's Big Boy was the second largest restaurant chain in the world, raking in $200 million a year—Howard Johnson's was first on the list, while McDonald's sat down at number three. Bob Wian built his last Big Boy in 1964, and today many of the original restaurants have been sold and converted to other restaurants.

As the fifties rolled around, popularity of the drive-in restaurant was at an all-time high. Customers seeking speed and convenience with their meals could just pull their cars into a stall and the food would be brought out to them, usually on a tray that hooked over the rolled-down window. The McDonald brothers had a drive-in in 1948 in San Bernardino. That was the first McDonald's, and it was racking up annual receipts of $200,000. There were many others too: Sonic, Blackies, Porky's, and a place called Mel's, made famous in the movie "American Graffiti."

But, as America entered the sixties, problems plagued the drive-in. Loud, rock-and-roll playing teenagers, looking for some action and a place to hang out, began overwhelming the parking lots. The cars that had pulled into the stalls would stay there as the youngsters socialized, keeping the paying customers away. The drive-ins had become tiny traffic jams of hormonally overwhelmed teens cruising for a date. The families looking to go out for a quick, quiet bite to eat could no longer enjoy the experience. Soon, under government pressure, practically all of the 2000 or so drive-ins in the country were shut down.

Meanwhile, the restaurant boom was shifting into fifth gear. Shoney's emerged in 1947 as a franchise of the Big Boy chain, then later would spin off on its own. In 1953, Danny's Donuts opened and eventually evolved into Denny's. The first International House of Pancakes opened its doors in 1958, around the same time a fresh new concept called Sizzler came onto the scene. Sizzler was an affordable steakhouse that combined sit-down dining with fast-food service. You'd order your steak at the front counter and then wait for your number to be called to pick it up. When you had your meal you'd find a seat in the dining room and eat as you would in a full-service restaurant.

In 1965, the face of casual dining would change significantly with the opening of the first T.G.I. Friday's in New York City. The restaurant was initially designed as a place for singles to meet, and was so popular that police had to build barricades around the restaurant to control the crowds. Soon this concept of the upbeat,

TOP 10 RESTAURANT COMPANIES

Rank	Company	Fiscal '95 Sales ($MM)
1.	**PepsIco, Inc.** (Pizza Hut, Taco Bell, KFC, Hot 'N Now, Chevy's, Eastside Mario's)	9,202.0
2.	**McDonald's Corp.** (McDonald's)	4,474.0
3.	**Darden Restaurants, Inc.** (Red Lobster, Olive Garden, Bahama Breeze)	3,200.0
4.	**Flagstar Cos. Inc.** (Denny's, Hardees, Quincy's, El Pollo Loco)	2,381.0
5.	**Wendy's International** (Wendy's Old-Fashioned Hamburgers)	1,416.3
6.	**Imasco Ltd.** (Hardees, Roy Rogers)	1,300.0
7.	**Brinker International** (Chili's, Romano's Macaroni Grill, On the Border)	1,160.0
8.	**Family Restaurants** (Chi-Chi's, El Torito, Coco's, Carrows, Reuben's, Jojos)	1,134.0
9.	**Little Caesar's** (Little Caesar's Pizza)	1,000.0
10.	**Metromedia** (Bennigan's, Ponderosa, Steak & Ale, Bonanza Family Grill)	986.0

Source: Nation's Restaurant News

entertaining atmosphere would be imitated the country over, and casual dining would get a huge shot in the tush.

When the first Hard Rock Cafe opened in London in 1971, a new trend emerged. With donated sequined jackets, gold records, and guitars hanging from the walls, this restaurant incorporated rock-and-roll nostalgia into its design. It wasn't enough to go to a restaurant just for food anymore, now people looked to be entertained. Surprisingly, it took twenty years for the trend to really mushroom. In 1991, the first Planet Hollywood opened in New York just down the street from the New York Hard Rock Cafe. Planet Hollywood was essentially the Hard Rock concept, with a Hollywood twist. Instead of displaying music memorabilia, Planet Hollywood is decorated with props and costumes from movies and television.

The smashing success of these "theme restaurants" created a surge of openings in the nineties. Today, in addition to the Hard Rock Cafe and Planet Hollywood, we have the Official All-Star Cafe, The Harley Davidson Cafe, The Motown Cafe, The Fashion Cafe, Dive!, House of Blues, and the NASCAR cafe, with several other new concepts in the pipeline.

The Crystal Ball

Restaurants have come a long way since the days of Happy Joseph's Nile Inn. Since the number of restaurants opening their doors is increasing every day at a phenomenal rate, so is the competition. To keep up, these full-service chains are having to overhaul menus on a regular basis. Gone are the days when owners could only change their menus once a year. Today menu items are added and dropped as often as every two months, and new concepts for food must constantly be explored. Many of these chains find they need to remodel their restaurants every five to seven years to stay fresh and interesting, and to hold onto their loyal customer base.

We're likely to see more restaurants developed with a heavy dose of fun and entertainment as a main component. In a recent survey, 44 percent of those polled said they want an upbeat entertaining atmosphere in the restaurants they frequent. That's probably why we're seeing numerous new concepts for theme restaurants similar to House of Blues, Dive!, or Planet Hollywood, and successful restaurants with a friendly, party-like atmosphere such as Applebee's, T.G.I. Friday's, and Red Robin.

With the recent dietary concerns regarding calories and fat intake, most of these chains have included special choices on their menus under headings like "Guiltless Grill," "Low-Fat and Fabulous," and "Lightside." The dishes usually include grilled chicken, pastas, and salads. It's a sure bet that we'll see more of this trend as restaurant chains unveil new dishes developed with health-conscious eaters in mind.

As long as we have to sustain our biological need for food, and because we are part of a society constantly craving speed, convenience, and entertainment, restaurants in America will flourish. Just exactly what new trends might develop in the future as restaurants continue to duke it out for our dining dollars is anyone's guess. The battlefield is littered with failures of one of the country's most competitive and cutthroat industries. If Happy Joe were in the business today, he might not be so happy.

But, who knows, he might have made millions sparking a trend in gazelle butt sandwiches. Think about it—drive-thru outlets dotting the globe, all with big neon signs off the highways bearing his infamous slogan: "Eat at Joe's. Get Your Butt Over Here, Now!"

Hmmm . . .

✳ Applebee's Quesadillas

Serves 1 or 2 as an appetizer

Menu Description: "Two cheeses, bacon, tomatoes, onions & jalapenos grilled between tortillas with guacamole, sour cream & salsa."

When Bill and T.J. Palmer opened their first restaurant in Atlanta, Georgia, in 1980, they realized their dream of building a full-service, reasonably-priced restaurant in a neighborhood setting. They called their first place T.J. Applebee's Edibles & Elixirs, and soon began franchising the concept. In 1988 some franchisees bought the rights to the name and changed it to Applebee's Neighborhood Grill & Bar. By that time, there were 54 restaurants in the organization. Today there are over 650, making Applebee's one of the fastest-growing restaurant chains in the world.

According to waiters at the restaurant, the easy-to-make and slightly spicy quesadillas are one of the most popular appetizers on the Applebee's menu. The recipe calls for 10-inch or "burrito-size" flour tortillas, which can be found in most supermarkets, but any size can be used in a pinch. Look for the jalapeño "nacho slices" in the ethnic or Mexican food section of the supermarket. You'll find these in jars or cans. Cilantro, which is growing immensely in popularity, can be found in the produce section near the parsley, and is also called fresh coriander or Chinese parsley.

2 **10-inch ("burrito-size") flour tortillas**
2 **tablespoons butter, softened**
⅓ **cup shredded Monterey Jack cheese**
⅓ **cup shredded Cheddar cheese**

½ **medium tomato, chopped**
2 **teaspoons diced onion**
1 **teaspoon diced canned jalapeño ("nacho slices")**
1 **slice bacon, cooked**
¼ **teaspoon finely chopped fresh cilantro**
Dash salt

On the side

Sour cream
Guacamole

Salsa

24

1. Heat a large frying pan over medium heat.
2. Spread half of the butter on one side of each tortilla. Put one tortilla, butter side down, in the hot pan.
3. Spread the cheeses evenly onto the center of the tortilla in the pan. You don't have to spread the cheese all the way to the edge. Leave a margin of an inch or so all the way around.

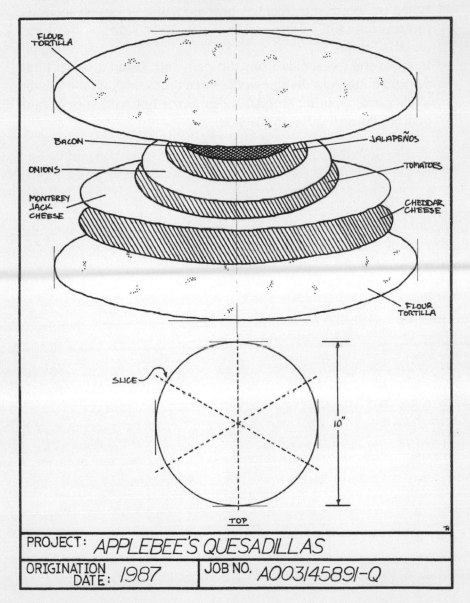

FLOUR TORTILLA

BACON

ONIONS

MONTEREY JACK CHEESE

JALAPEÑOS

TOMATOES

CHEDDAR CHEESE

FLOUR TORTILLA

SLICE

10"

TOP

PROJECT: *APPLEBEE'S QUESADILLAS*

ORIGINATION DATE: *1987*

JOB NO. *A003145891-Q*

4. Sprinkle the tomato, onion, and jalapeño over the cheese.
5. Crumble the slice of cooked bacon and sprinkle it over the other ingredients.
6. Sprinkle the cilantro and a dash of salt over the other ingredients.
7. Top off the quesadilla with the remaining tortilla, being sure that the buttered side is facing up.
8. When the bottom tortilla has browned, after 45 to 90 seconds, flip the quesadilla over and grill the other side for the same length of time.
9. Remove the quesadilla from the pan, and, using a sharp knife or pizza cutter, cut the quesadilla three times through the middle like a pizza, creating 6 equal slices. Serve hot with sour cream, guacamole, and salsa on the side.

✳ Applebee's Pizza Sticks

Serves 6 to 8 as an appetizer

Menu Description: **"Parmesan:** Thin crusty strips of pizza dough topped with herbs & melted Italian cheese, served with marinara sauce.
Loaded: Add Italian sausage & pepperoni."

Each Applebee's makes an effort to decorate the inside of the restaurant with pictures and memorabilia from the neighborhood in which it is located. You'll see photographs of local heroes and students, license plates, banners, old souvenirs, trinkets, and an-tiques—all representing area history. Take a look around the walls of the next Applebee's you visit. Maybe you can find something you lost several years ago.

Meanwhile, here's a find: pizza sticks that are made from dough that is proofed, fried, and then broiled. The frying adds a unique flavor and texture to the dough that you won't get with traditional pizza. I've designed this recipe to use the premade dough that comes in tubes (you know, like the stuff from that dough boy). But you can make this with any dough recipe you might like, or with one from this book (which I know you'll like, see page 211). Just roll the dough into a 10 × 15-inch rectangle before slicing.

These appetizers can be made either in the Parmesan version without meat, or "loaded" with sausage and pepperoni. This recipe yields a lot, so it makes good party food.

Marinara Dipping Sauce

1 8-ounce can tomato sauce	½ teaspoon dried oregano
1 tomato, chopped	
1 tablespoon diced onion	⅛ teaspoon salt
1 teaspoon sugar	⅛ teaspoon dried basil

Parmesan Pizza Sticks

1 10-ounce tube instant pizza dough (Pillsbury is good)

2 to 4 cups vegetable oil for frying

1¾ cups grated mozzarella cheese

¼ cup grated fresh Parmesan cheese

½ teaspoon dried oregano

¼ teaspoon dried basil

¼ teaspoon caraway seeds

¼ teaspoon garlic salt

Optional (for the "Loaded")

3 ounces pepperoni, diced

3 ounces Italian sausage, cooked and crumbled

1. Preheat the oven to 425 degrees F.
2. Prepare the dipping sauce by combining all of the marinara ingredients in a small, uncovered saucepan and bringing the mixture to a boil. Reduce the heat, cover, and simmer the sauce for ½ hour. (The sauce can be made ahead and kept, refrigerated, for several days.)
3. Prepare the pizza sticks by first proofing the dough. Unroll the dough onto a cutting board and straighten the edges. It should form a rectangle that is longer from left to right than top to bottom. With a sharp knife or pizza cutter, slice through the middle of the dough lengthwise. This will divide the rectangle into two thinner rectangles that will measure 4 to 5 inches from top to bottom.
4. Slice the dough from top to bottom into 1½-inch-wide pieces. You should have somewhere between 20 and 24 dough slices.
5. Place the slices onto a greased cookie sheet about ½ inch apart and bake for 3 minutes. You may have to use more than one cookie sheet. This will proof the dough so that it becomes stiff.
6. Heat vegetable oil in a frying pan or deep fryer to 350 degrees F. Oil should be at least ½ inch deep if using a stovetop pan. You will want to use more oil with a deep fryer.
7. Fry pizza sticks 5 to 6 at a time for about 1 minute per side or until they are a dark golden brown. Remove them from the oil onto a cloth or paper towel to drain.

8. When all the pizza dough sticks are fried, arrange them once again on the cookie sheet(s). You may want to line the cookie sheets with foil to make cleanup easier. Preheat the broiler.
9. Sprinkle the mozzarella cheese evenly over the dough.
10. Sprinkle the Parmesan cheese evenly over the mozzarella.

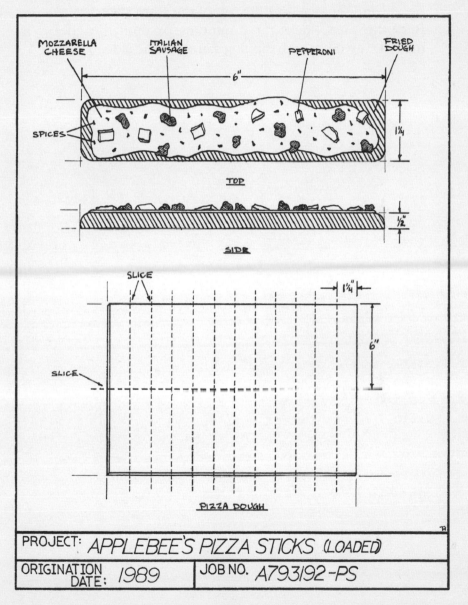

29

11. Combine the oregano, basil, caraway seeds, and garlic salt in a small bowl. If your oregano and basil are fairly coarse you can use your thumb and first finger to crunch the spice up a little, making it a finer blend.
12. Sprinkle the spice mixture over the cheese.
13. If you want to make the "loaded" variety, sprinkle the pepperoni and sausage over the top of the pizza sticks.
14. Broil the pizza sticks for 2 minutes or until the cheese is melted. Serve hot with dipping sauce on the side.

✳ Applebee's Oriental Chicken Salad

Serves 1 as an entree (can be doubled)

Menu Description: "Crisp Oriental greens topped with chunks of crunchy Chicken Fingers, toasted almonds & crispy rice noodles tossed in a light Oriental vinaigrette."

Applebee's 60-item menu is revised at least twice a year. That means about 40 percent of the entire menu changes on a regular basis, with those selections varying from location to location. The other 60 percent are items found on menus in all of the Applebee's restaurants, and they seldom change. This practice of constant menu retooling is becoming more frequent in all of the large restaurant chains these days. As competition grows, the chains find they must alter their menus regularly to keep discriminating customers interested.

Even though the Oriental Chicken Salad, which is considered one of the restaurant's signature items, has been on the menu for some time now, it's possible that by the time you are reading this book it has been replaced by another salad selection. If that happens, here's the only way you can still enjoy this salad creation—by making your own. You'll love the Oriental dressing with the unique, nutty flavor of roasted sesame oil. This type of oil is becoming quite popular today and can be found in the supermarket near the other oils or where the Asian food is displayed.

Oriental Dressing

3 tablespoons honey
1½ tablespoons white vinegar
4 teaspoons mayonnaise

1 tablespoon Grey Poupon Dijon mustard
⅛ teaspoon sesame oil

31

Salad

2 to 4 cups vegetable oil for frying	3 cups chopped romaine lettuce
1 egg	1 cup chopped red cabbage
½ cup milk	1 cup chopped napa cabbage
½ cup all-purpose flour	½ carrot, julienned or shredded
½ cup cornflake crumbs	1 green onion, sliced
1 teaspoon salt	1 tablespoon sliced almonds
¼ teaspoon pepper	⅓ cup chow mein noodles
1 boneless, skinless chicken breast half	

1. Using an electric mixer, blend together all the ingredients for the dressing in a small bowl. Put the dressing in the refrigerator to chill while you prepare the salad.
2. Preheat the oil in a deep fryer or frying pan over medium heat. You want the temperature of the oil to be around 350 degrees F. If using a frying pan, the oil should be around ½ inch deep. More oil can be used in a deep fryer so that the chicken is immersed.
3. In a small, shallow bowl beat the egg, add the milk, and mix well.
4. In another bowl, combine the flour with the cornflake crumbs, salt, and pepper.
5. Cut the chicken breast into 4 or 5 long strips. Dip each strip of chicken first into the egg mixture then into the flour mixture, coating each piece completely.
6. Fry each chicken finger for 5 minutes or until the coating has darkened to brown.
7. Prepare the salad by tossing the romaine with the red cabbage, napa cabbage, and carrot.
8. Sprinkle the green onion on top of the lettuce mixture.
9. Sprinkle the almonds over the salad, then the chow mein noodles.
10. Cut the chicken into bite-size chunks. Place the chicken on the salad, forming a pile in the middle. Serve with the salad dressing on the side.

✳ Applebee's Club House Grill

Serves 1 as an entree (can be doubled)

Menu Description: "Applebee's signature hot club sandwich with warm sliced ham & turkey, Cheddar, tomatoes, mayonnaise & Bar-B-Que sauce on thick-sliced grilled French bread. Served with a side of coleslaw."

Here's a sandwich which Applebee's claims is a signature item for the chain. I can see why—it's creative, yet simple. And pretty tasty. It's a cross between a club sandwich and a grilled cheese. So, if you like both of those, you'll love this. And it helps that the sandwich is easy to make when you're as lazy as I am.

For the sliced turkey and ham, go to your deli service counter in the supermarket and get the stuff they machine-slice real thin for sandwiches. This usually tastes the best. If you don't have a service counter, you can find the thin-sliced meats prepackaged near the hot dogs and bologna.

2 **thick slices French bread**	2 **slices deli-sliced turkey breast**
1 **tablespoon butter, softened**	2 **slices deli-sliced ham**
2 **teaspoons mayonnaise**	2 **slices tomato**
⅓ **cup shredded Cheddar cheese**	2 **teaspoons barbecue sauce (Bullseye is best)**

1. Spread the butter evenly over one side of each slice of bread.
2. Put one slice of bread, butter side down, into a preheated frying pan over medium heat.
3. Spread the mayonnaise over the unbuttered side of the grilling bread.
4. Sprinkle half of the Cheddar cheese over the mayonnaise.
5. Lay the turkey and ham in the pan next to the bread for about 30 seconds to heat it up.
6. When it's warm, lay the turkey on the cheese.
7. Place the tomato slices on the turkey.
8. Spread the barbecue sauce over the tomato slices.
9. Lay the ham on the tomatoes.
10. Sprinkle the remainder of the cheese over the ham.
11. Top off the sandwich with the other slice of bread, being sure that the buttered side is facing up.

12. By now the first side of bread should be golden brown. Flip the sandwich over and grill the other side for 2 to 3 minutes or until golden brown as well.
13. Remove the sandwich from the pan and cut in half diagonally. Serve with additional barbecue sauce on the side.

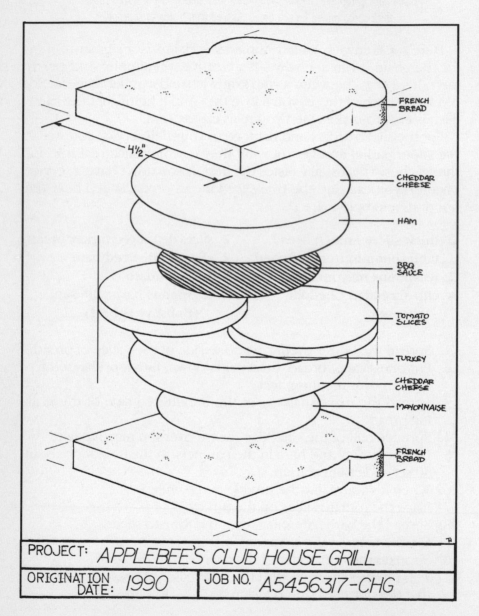

FRENCH BREAD

4½"

CHEDDAR CHEESE

HAM

BBQ SAUCE

TOMATO SLICES

TURKEY

CHEDDAR CHEESE

MAYONNAISE

FRENCH BREAD

PROJECT: APPLEBEE'S CLUB HOUSE GRILL

ORIGINATION DATE: 1990   JOB NO. A5456317-CHG

✳ Applebee's Tijuana "Philly" Steak Sandwich

Serves 1 as an entree (can be doubled)

Menu Description: "Lean shaved 'Philly' steak folded into a grilled tortilla roll with Monterey Jack & Cheddar, sautéed mushrooms, onions, tomatoes, bacon & jalapeños."

With the acquisition of 13 Rio Bravo Cantinas in 1994, Applebee's made its move into the competitive "Mexican casual dining sector." Perhaps it's the company's interest in Mexican food that inspired this Philadelphia-Tijuana hybrid sandwich. The steak, cheese, mushrooms, and onions give the sandwich a Philly taste, while the tomatoes, bacon, jalapeños, and the tortilla take you across the border.

I really like this newer addition to the menu, probably because I'm a big cheese-steak fan who also loves Mexican food. As you can see from this dish and the one before it, Applebee's has a knack for breathing new life into old sandwich concepts. I hope you'll find this one worth a try.

You shouldn't have any trouble locating the ingredients, except maybe the cilantro. It's becoming very popular so hopefully it will be easy to find. Just look in the produce section near the parsley, where it might also be called fresh coriander or Chinese parsley (not to be confused with Italian parsley). *¡Muy bien!*

1 mushroom, diced
1 tablespoon plus ½ teaspoon butter, softened
Salt
Pepper
3 ounces chipped beef *or* 1½ slices Steak-Umm frozen sandwich steaks
¼ cup shredded Cheddar cheese
¼ cup shredded Monterey Jack cheese
1 10-inch ("burrito-size") flour tortilla
1 heaping tablespoon diced tomato
1 teaspoon diced red onion
¼ teaspoon finely chopped fresh cilantro
1 slice bacon, cooked

35

On the Side

Shredded lettuce
Sour cream

Salsa

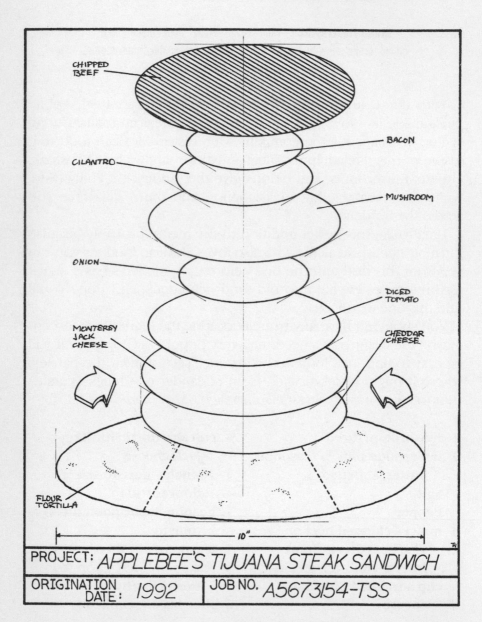

CHIPPED BEEF

BACON

CILANTRO

MUSHROOM

ONION

DICED TOMATO

MONTEREY JACK CHEESE

CHEDDAR CHEESE

FLOUR TORTILLA

10"

PROJECT: *APPLEBEE'S TIJUANA STEAK SANDWICH*

ORIGINATION DATE: *1992*   JOB NO. *A5673154-TSS*

36

1. Sauté the mushroom in a small pan with ½ teaspoon butter and a dash of salt and pepper. The mushroom pieces should start to turn brown when they are done.
2. Break or cut the beef into bite-size pieces and grill it in another pan over medium heat until brown. Add a dash of salt and pepper. Drain off the fat.
3. Build your sandwich by first sprinkling both cheeses into the center of the tortilla. Keep in mind when adding the cheese that you will be folding in the sides like a burrito, so leave some room on each side.
4. Sprinkle the tomato, onion, sautéed mushroom, and cilantro over the cheese.
5. Crumble the bacon and sprinkle it over the cheese as well.
6. Sprinkle the cooked beef over the other ingredients, then add a bit more salt and pepper, if desired.
7. Fold the sides in, then use the 1 tablespoon butter to butter the top and bottom of the "sandwich" and grill it in a hot pan over medium heat for 2 minutes per side, or until the tortilla becomes golden brown and the cheese is melted.
8. Slice the "sandwich" in half diagonally and serve hot on a plate with shredded lettuce, sour cream, and salsa on the side.

✳ Benihana Hibachi
Chicken and Hibachi Steak

Serves 3 to 4 as an entree

When 20-year-old Rocky Aoki came to New York City from Japan with his wrestling team in 1959 he was convinced it was the land of opportunity. Just five years later he used $10,000 he had saved plus another $20,000 that he borrowed to open a Benihana steakhouse on the West Side of Manhattan. His concept of bringing the chefs out from the back kitchen to prepare the food in front of customers on a specially designed hibachi grill was groundbreaking. The restaurant was such a smashing success that it paid for itself within six months.

The most popular items at the restaurant are the Hibachi Chicken and Hibachi Steak, which are prepared at your table on an open hibachi grill. But, since most home kitchens are not fitted with a hibachi grill, you'll have to improvise. You will likely have to use two pans; one for the meat and mushrooms, and the other for the remaining vegetables. And since many of today's cooking surfaces are coated with scratchable, nonstick coatings, we won't be slicing the meat and vegetables while they are sizzling on the hot cooking surface as the Benihana chefs do. Nor will you be required to flip a mushroom into your hat.

4 boneless, skinless chicken breast halves	4 tablespoons butter
	Salt
1 large onion	Pepper
2 medium zucchini	2 teaspoons lemon juice
2 cups sliced mushrooms	3 teaspoons sesame seeds
2 tablespoons vegetable oil	6 cups bean sprouts
6 tablespoons soy sauce	

On the Side

Mustard Sauce (page 41)
Ginger Sauce (page 42)

38

1. Before you begin cooking be sure that the chicken, onion, zucchini, and mushrooms have been sliced into bite-size pieces. For the onion, slice it as if you were making onion rings, then quarter those slices. For the zucchini, first slice them into long, thin strips, then cut across those strips four or five times to make bite-size pieces that are 1 to 1½ inches long.
2. Spread 1 tablespoon of oil in a large frying pan over medium/high heat. Spread another tablespoon of oil in another pan over medium/high heat.
3. Begin by sautéing the sliced chicken in one of the pans. Add 1 tablespoon of soy sauce, 1 tablespoon of butter, and a dash of salt and pepper to the chicken.
4. Add the onion and zucchini to the other pan. Add 2 tablespoons soy sauce, 1 tablespoon butter, and a dash of salt and pepper. Sauté the vegetables as long as the chicken is cooking, being sure to stir both pans often.
5. When the chicken has sautéed for about 2 minutes or when it appears white on all sides, slide the meat to one side of the pan, pour lemon juice on it, then add the mushrooms to the other side of the pan. Pour 1 tablespoon of the soy sauce over the mushrooms, then add 1 tablespoon of butter plus a dash of salt and pepper. Continue to stir both pans.
6. After 6 to 8 minutes, or when the chicken is done, sprinkle 1 teaspoon of sesame seeds over the chicken, then mix the chicken with the mushrooms. Spoon the chicken mixture in four even portions on four plates next to four even portions of the vegetables from the other pan.
7. Pour the bean sprouts into the same pan in which you cooked the vegetables, and cook over high heat. Add 2 tablespoons soy sauce, 1 tablespoon butter, and a dash of salt and pepper.
8. Cook the sprouts for only a minute or two, or until they have tenderized. Just before you serve the sprouts, sprinkle 2 teaspoons of sesame seeds on them. Serve the sprouts next to the chicken and vegetables with mustard sauce and ginger sauce on the side.

Hibachi Steak

You can also make a Hibachi Steak like you would find at the restaurant. Just follow the chicken recipe, substituting a 16-ounce sirloin steak for the chicken. Also eliminate the lemon juice and sesame seeds from the recipe.

Keep in mind that your sliced beef will likely cook in half the time of the chicken, depending on how rare you like it.

✳ Benihana
Dipping Sauces

Makes ⅔ cup of each sauce

The origin of the name of this chain of Japanese steakhouses dates back to 1935. That's when founder Rocky Aoki's father, Yunosuke Aoki, opened a small coffee shop in Japan and named it "Benihana" after a wild red flower that grew near the front door of his shop. Next time you're at Benihana, look carefully and you'll notice that bright red flower has been incorporated into the restaurant's logo.

With most of the cooking performed before your eyes on an open hibachi grill, Benihana maintains a much smaller kitchen than most restaurants, allowing practically the entire restaurant to become productive, money-generating dining space. The limited space behind the scenes is for storage, office and dressing rooms, and a small preparation area for noncooked items like these sauces. Use them to dip food in—like the Hibachi Steak or Chicken (pages 38 and 39). These sauces will go well with a variety of Asian dishes and can be frozen in sealed containers for weeks at a time.

Mustard Sauce (for chicken and beef)

¼ cup soy sauce
¼ cup water
2 teaspoons Oriental mustard*

2 teaspoons heavy cream
½ teaspoon garlic powder

Combine all of the ingredients in a small bowl and mix until well combined. Chill before serving.

*Can be found in the international or Asian food section of your supermarket.

Ginger Sauce (for vegetables and seafood)

¼ cup chopped onion
¼ cup soy sauce
1 clove garlic, minced
½ ounce gingerroot (a nickel-size slice), peeled and chopped

Juice of ½ lemon (2 tablespoons)
½ teaspoon sugar
¼ teaspoon white vinegar

Combine all of the ingredients in a blender and blend on low speed for 30 seconds or until the gingerroot and garlic have been puréed. Chill before serving.

✳ Benihana Japanese Fried Rice

Serves 4 as a side dish

The talented chefs at Benihana cook food on hibachi grills with flair and charisma, treating the preparation like a tiny stage show. They juggle salt and pepper shakers, trim food with lightning speed, and flip shrimp and mushrooms perfectly onto serving plates or into their tall chef's hat.

One of the side dishes that everyone seems to love is the fried rice. At Benihana this dish is prepared by chefs with precooked rice on open hibachi grills, and is ordered à la carte to complement any Benihana entree, including Hibachi Steak and Chicken. I like when the rice is thrown onto the hot hibachi grill and seems to come alive as it sizzles and dances around like a bunch of little jumping beans. Okay, so I'm easily amused.

This version of that popular side dish will go well with just about any Japanese entree and can be partially prepared ahead of time, and kept in the refrigerator until the rest of the meal is close to done (check out the "Tidbits").

1 **cup uncooked long grain converted or parboiled rice (*not* instant or quick white rice)**	½ **cup diced onion (½ small onion)**
2 **eggs, beaten**	1½ **tablespoons butter**
1 **cup frozen peas, thawed**	2 **tablespoons soy sauce**
2 **tablespoons finely grated carrot**	**Salt**
	Pepper

1. Cook the rice following the instructions on the package. This should take about 20 minutes. Pour the rice into a large bowl to let it cool.
2. Scramble the eggs in a small pan over medium heat. Chop scrambled chunks of egg into small pea-size bits with your spatula while cooking.
3. When the rice has cooled, add the peas, carrot, eggs, and onion to the bowl. Carefully toss all of the ingredients together.
4. Melt the butter in a large frying pan over medium/high heat.

5. When the butter has completely melted, dump the rice mixture into the pan and add the soy sauce plus a dash of salt and pepper. Cook the rice mixture for 6 to 8 minutes, stirring often.

Tidbits

This fried rice can be prepared ahead of time by cooking the rice, then adding the peas, carrot, and scrambled egg plus half of the soy sauce. Keep this refrigerated until you are ready to fry it in the butter. That's when you add the salt, pepper, and remaining soy sauce.

✳ Bennigan's Buffalo Chicken Sandwich

Serves 1 as an entree (can be doubled)

Menu Description: "Our spicy sauce tops a tender, fried, marinated chicken breast. Served with a tangy bleu cheese dressing."

When the first Bennigan's opened in Atlanta, Georgia, in 1976, it resembled an Irish pub. The green decor with brass accents, the Irish-style memorabilia hanging on the walls, and the upbeat friendly atmosphere made the establishment extremely popular, especially during St. Patrick's Day celebrations. Originally, the restaurant was best known for the bar, which served tasty appetizers and creative drinks, but that has since changed. As the restaurant chain expanded across the country, its menu grew to more than 50 items, making 220-outlet Bennigan's a popular casual dining stop.

If you're a big buffalo wings fan, as I am, you'll really dig this sandwich that puts the zest flavor of hot wings between two buns. This recent addition to the Bennigan's menu has become a popular pick for the lunch or dinner crowd that likes its food on the spicy side. Feel free to double the recipe, but fry the chicken breasts one at a time.

Oil for deep-frying	1 hamburger bun
½ cup all-purpose flour	1 leaf green leaf lettuce
½ teaspoon salt	2 slices tomato
½ cup whole milk	1 slice red onion
1 boneless, skinless chicken breast half	2 tablespoons Louisiana Hot Sauce or Frank's Red Hot

On the Side

Bleu cheese dressing

1. Preheat the oil to 350 degrees F in a deep fryer or a large frying pan over medium heat. Use just enough oil to cover the chicken breast.
2. Stir together the flour and salt in a medium bowl. Pour the milk into another medium bowl.

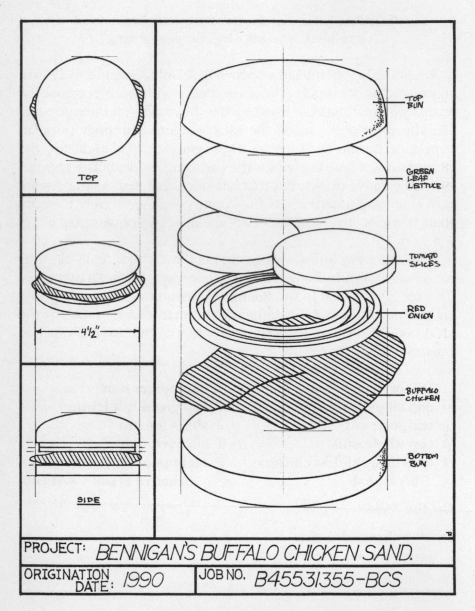

TOP

4½"

SIDE

TOP BUN

GREEN LEAF LETTUCE

TOMATO SLICES

RED ONION

BUFFALO CHICKEN

BOTTOM BUN

PROJECT: BENNIGAN'S BUFFALO CHICKEN SAND.

ORIGINATION DATE: 1990   JOB NO. B45531355-BCS

3. Trim the chicken of any fat. Cut the thin, pointed end off the breast. Pound on the chicken with a meat-tenderizing mallet to flatten the breast and shape it to fit better on the bun.
4. Dip the chicken in milk, then in the flour, being sure to coat the entire surface of the chicken. Take the coated chicken breast and repeat the process. Let the chicken sit in the refrigerator for 10 to 15 minutes.
5. Drop the chicken breast into the hot oil and fry for 10 minutes or until the outside becomes golden brown. Drain on paper towels.
6. As the chicken is frying, toast or grill the face of the hamburger bun until light brown.
7. The sandwich is served open face, so place the bun face up on the plate. On the face of the top bun place the leaf of lettuce.
8. On the lettuce stack two slices of tomato.
9. Separate the slice of red onion and place 2 to 3 rings of onion on the tomato slices.
10. When the chicken breast has cooked and drained, place it in a plastic container that has a lid. Pour the hot sauce into the container, put the lid on top, and shake gently to coat the chicken with hot sauce. Be sure to shake only enough to coat the chicken. If you shake too hard, the crispy coating will fall off the chicken.
11. Stack the chicken breast on the bottom half of the hamburger bun and place it on the plate beside the top half of the sandwich. Serve open face, with bleu cheese dressing on the side.

✳ Bennigan's California Turkey Sandwich

Serves 1 as an entree (can be doubled)

Menu Description: "Sliced turkey, avocado, tomato, sprouts, and lettuce with mayonnaise on wheat bread."

The successful chain of Bennigan's restaurants is owned by Metromedia, one of the largest privately held partnerships in the country. Metromedia ranks second on the list of the country's largest casual dining restaurant companies, just behind Little Caesar's Pizza. Other restaurant chains controlled by Metromedia include Steak and Ale, Montana Steak Company, Ponderosa Steakhouse, and Bonanza Steakhouse chains. Altogether Metromedia owns more than 1500 restaurants that ring up nearly half a billion dollars in revenue each year.

It's funny how any sandwich with avocados, sprouts, tomatoes, and lettuce in it winds up with "California" somewhere in the name. This recipe is not exactly a healthier alternative with all the mayonnaise and avocado in there, but if it's low-fat you're looking for, simply substitute a "light" mayonnaise for the regular stuff, ditch the avocado, and you're on your way to the beach.

2 slices wheat bread	½ cup alfalfa sprouts
1 tablespoon mayonnaise	1 leaf green leaf lettuce
¼ pound deli-sliced turkey breast	½ small avocado
2 slices tomato	Salt

1. Spread ½ tablespoon of mayonnaise on one face of each slice of bread.
2. Assemble the sandwich by stacking the turkey on the mayonnaise side of one slice of bread.
3. Place the tomato slices on the turkey.
4. Arrange the sprouts on top of the tomato slices.
5. Place the lettuce leaf on the sprouts.
6. Slice the avocado into thin slices and arrange the slices on the lettuce.

48

7. Top off the sandwich by placing a slice of bread, mayo side down, on the avocado.
8. Cut the sandwich twice, diagonally from corner to corner, making four triangular pieces.
9. Stick a toothpick straight down through the middle of each sandwich piece to hold it together.

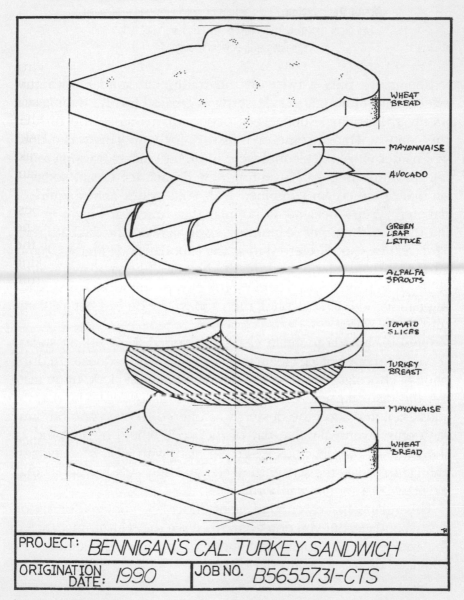

WHEAT BREAD

MAYONNAISE

AVOCADO

GREEN LEAF LETTUCE

ALFALFA SPROUTS

TOMATO SLICES

TURKEY BREAST

MAYONNAISE

WHEAT BREAD

PROJECT: BENNIGAN'S CAL. TURKEY SANDWICH

ORIGINATION DATE: 1990   JOB NO. B565573I-CTS

49

✳ Bennigan's Cookie Mountain Sundae

Serves 6 to 7

Menu Description: "Four scoops of vanilla ice cream between
two giant chocolate chip cookies. Drizzled with hot fudge and
sprinkled with powdered sugar."

Bennigan's puts a twist on the traditional sundae with this
sweet treat. Although this dessert was created for the Bennigan's
menu, the original sundae has been with us since the turn of
the century. Here's some cool history for you: This was a time
when alternatives to alcohol were in high demand, so soda fountain proprietors began inventing new drinks. Ice cream sodas—
scoops of ice cream combined with soda water and a squirt of
flavored syrup—became so popular that Americans were enjoy-
ing them to the point of gluttony, especially on the Sabbath day.
The treat was soon referred to as the "Sunday Soda Menace," and
after Evanston, Illinois, became the first city to enact laws against
selling ice cream sodas (shame!), the new prohibition was spreading nationwide. First alcohol, then sodas . . . you can bet a substitute was in order.

One day a soda fountain clerk, prohibited from selling sodas,
served up a bowl of ice cream to a customer who requested a drib-
bling of chocolate syrup on the top. The fountain clerk, upon tast-
ing the dish himself, found that he had discovered a new taste
sensation, and soon the dessert was offered to everyone on Sun-
days only. Eventually that day of the week would be adopted as
the name of the delicious ice-cream dish, with a bit of a spelling
change to satisfy the scrutinizing clergy. The "soda-less soda" that
we now call a sundae was born.

This recipe makes enough giant chocolate cookies for six or
seven sundaes, but you don't have to serve them all at once. Store
the cookies in an airtight container and assemble the sundaes as
you need them . . . on any day of the week.

Chocolate Chip Cookies

½ cup softened butter
¼ cup granulated sugar
¾ cup packed brown sugar
1 egg
1 teaspoon vanilla
1¼ cups all-purpose flour

½ teaspoon salt
½ teaspoon baking powder
½ teaspoon baking soda
1 cup semisweet chocolate chips (6 ounces)

½ gallon vanilla ice cream
1 16-ounce jar hot fudge topping

Powdered sugar

1. Preheat the oven to 350 degrees F.
2. Make the cookies by creaming together the butter, sugars, egg, and vanilla in a medium-size bowl.
3. In a separate bowl, sift together the flour, salt, baking powder, and baking soda. Combine the dry ingredients with the butter mixture and mix well.
4. Add the chocolate chips and mix once more.
5. Roll the dough into golfball-size portions and place them 4 inches apart on an ungreased cookie sheet. With your hand, press down on the dough to flatten it to about ½ inch thick. You will likely have to use two cookie sheets for the 12 to 14 cookies the recipe will make. If you use the same cookie sheet for the second batch, be sure to let it cool before placing the dough on it.
6. Bake the cookies for 12 to 14 minutes or until they become a light shade of brown.
7. The cookies served with this dessert have a hole in the center so that when you pour on the hot fudge it flows down through the hole onto the ice cream in the middle. When you take the cookies out of the oven, use the opening of an empty glass soda or beer bottle like a cookie cutter to cut a 1-inch hole in the center of each cookie. Turn the bottle upside down and press the opening into the center of each cookie, rotating the bottle back and forth until the center of the cookie is cut out. Because the cookie centers will push into the bottle as you go, you'll have to rinse the bottle out before recycling. (If you

prefer, you can punch holes in just half of the cookies; these will be the cookies that are stacked on top of the ice cream.)

8. When the cookies have cooled, take four small scoops (about ¼ cup each) of ice cream and arrange them on the top of one cookie that has been placed in the center of the serving plate.

9. Place another cookie on top of the ice cream.

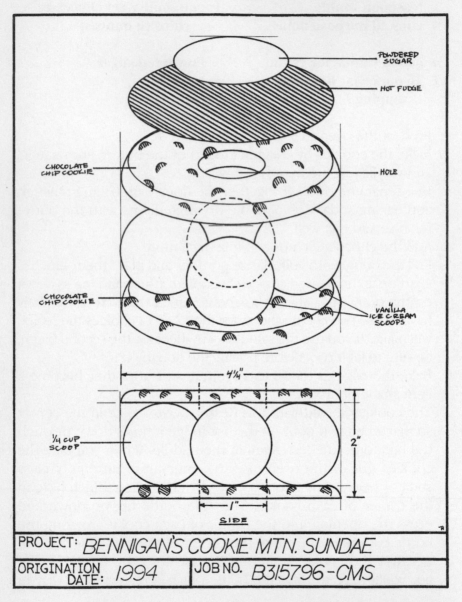

PROJECT: *BENNIGAN'S COOKIE MTN. SUNDAE*

ORIGINATION DATE: *1994*   JOB NO. *B315796-CMS*

10. Heat up the fudge in a microwave or in the top of a double boiler just long enough to soften the topping so that it is easy to pour. Pour 3 to 4 tablespoons of hot fudge over the top cookie. Let the fudge drizzle down the sides of the ice cream and through the hole that has been cut in the center of the top cookie.

11. Use a sifter or fine strainer to spread a dusting of powdered sugar onto the sundae and around the surface of the serving plate. Repeat with the remaining ingredients for the desired number of servings. The leftover ingredients (if any) can be saved for additional servings later.

✳ Big Boy Cream of Broccoli Soup

Serves 4 as an appetizer or 2 as an entree

Menu Description: *"Our famous Big Boy soups and chili are made fresh daily from fresh vegetables, pure cream and only the finest ingredients."*

In 1936, Bob Wian had to make the painful decision to sell his cherished 1933 DeSoto roadster to buy a ten-stool lunch counter from a pair of elderly ladies in Glendale, California. He named his new restaurant Bob's Pantry, and went to work behind the counter himself. Receipts from his first day totaled only twelve dollars. But with the creation of a new hamburger just the next year, and a name change to Bob's Big Boy, business took off. Within three years Bob had expanded his first store and built another location in Los Angeles. In 1948 Bob Wian was voted mayor of Glendale.

A cup of the broccoli soup makes a great first course or a nice partner to a sandwich. I first designed this recipe using frozen broccoli, but the frozen stuff just isn't as tasty as a big bunch of firm, fresh broccoli. So go shopping, and get chopping.

Served in a large bowl, this soup can be a small meal in itself, or it serves four as an appetizer. Try it with a pinch of shredded Cheddar cheese on top.

4 cups chicken broth	**¼ teaspoon salt**
1 large bunch broccoli, chopped (3 cups)	**Dash ground pepper**
	¼ cup all-purpose flour
½ cup diced onion	**2 ounces ham (⅓ cup diced)**
1 bay leaf	**½ cup heavy cream**

1. Combine the chicken broth, broccoli, onion, bay leaf, salt, and pepper in a large saucepan over high heat. When the broth comes to a boil, turn down the heat and simmer, covered, for 30 minutes. The vegetables will become tender.
2. Transfer a little more than half of the broth and vegetable mix-

ture to a blender or food processor. Mix on low speed for 20 to 30 seconds. This will finely chop the vegetables to nearly a purée. (Be careful blending hot liquids. You may want to let the mixture cool a bit before transferring and blending it.)

3. Pour the blended mixture back into the saucepan over medium/low heat. Add the flour and whisk until all lumps have dissolved.

4. Add the diced ham and the cream to the other ingredients and continue to simmer for 10 to 15 minutes or until the soup is as thick as you like it.

Tidbits

Because some ham is much saltier than others, I was conservative on the amount of salt in this recipe. You may find that you need more.

✳ Big Boy Original Double-Decker Hamburger Classic

Serves 1 as an entree (can be doubled)

Menu Description: "1/4 pound of 100% pure beef in two patties with American cheese, crisp lettuce and our special sauce on a sesame seed bun."

Bob Wian's little ten-stool diner, Bob's Pantry, was in business only a short time in Glendale, California, before establishing a following of regular customers—among them the band members from Chuck Foster's Orchestra. One February night in 1937, the band came by after a gig as they often did to order a round of burgers. In a playful mood, bass player Stewie Strange sat down on a stool and uttered, "How about something different for a change, Bob?" Bob thought it might be funny to play along and serve up Stewie a burger he could barely get his mouth around. So Bob cut a bun into three slices, rather than the usual two, and stacked on two hamburger patties along with lettuce, cheese, and his special sauce. When Stewie tasted the huge sandwich and loved it, every band member wanted his own!

Just a few days later, a plump little six-year-old named Richard Woodruff came into the diner and charmed Bob into letting him do odd jobs in exchange for a burger or two. He often wore baggy overalls and had an appetite that forced the affectionate nickname "Fat Boy."* Bob thought it was the perfect name for his new burger, except the name was already being used as a trademark for another product. So the name of the new burger, along with Bob's booming chain of restaurants, was changed to "Big Boy." The company's tradename Big Boy character is from a cartoonist's napkin sketch of "fat boy," little Richard Woodruff.

*Please understand that these are not my choice of words to describe young Richard Woodruff. I prefer the more socially sensitive terms: "Weight-blessed Adolescent," or "Young Adult with a Thinness Deficit." However, I do realize that neither of these descriptions would be a good name for a hamburger.

The Big Boy hamburger was the first of the double-decker hamburgers. McDonald's Big Mac, the world's best-known burger that came more than 30 years later, was inspired by Bob Wian's original creation. See if you can get your mouth around it.

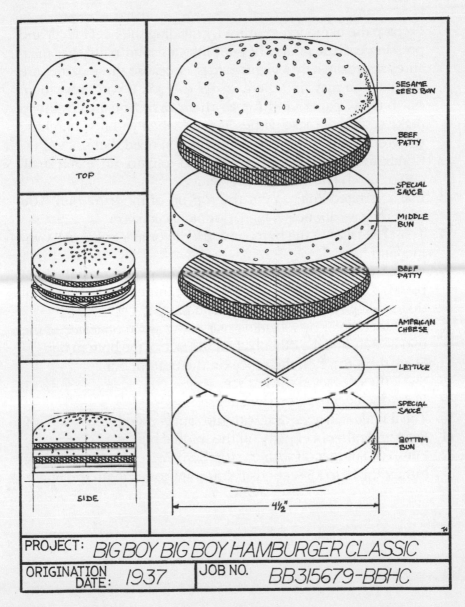

TOP

SIDE

SESAME SEED BUN

BEEF PATTY

SPECIAL SAUCE

MIDDLE BUN

BEEF PATTY

AMERICAN CHEESE

LETTUCE

SPECIAL SAUCE

BOTTOM BUN

4½"

PROJECT: *BIG BOY BIG BOY HAMBURGER CLASSIC*

ORIGINATION DATE: *1937*   JOB NO. *BB315679-BBHC*

¼ pound ground beef	Top half of additional
1½ tablespoons mayonnaise	hamburger bun
1 teaspoon relish	Salt
1 teaspoon tomato sauce	¼ cup shredded lettuce
1 sesame seed hamburger bun	1 slice American cheese

1. Prepare the hamburger patties by dividing the beef in half and pressing each ⅛ pound of beef into a round patty that measures approximately 4 inches across. Because these patties are so thin, you may find them easier to cook if you press them out on wax paper, and freeze them first. You may want to make several of these patties at once when you first purchase the ground beef, then cook them as you need them.

2. Combine the mayonnaise, relish, and tomato sauce in a small cup or bowl. This is the "secret sauce."

3. Use a serrated knife to cut the top off of the extra bun. You want to leave about a ½-inch, double-faced slice.

4. Toast the faces of the buns on a griddle or in a frying pan over medium heat.

5. When the buns are toasted, use the same pan to cook the beef patties. Cook the patties for about 2 minutes per side or until done, being sure to lightly salt each patty.

6. Build the burger by spreading half of the sauce on a face of the middle bun, and the other half on the face of the bottom bun.

7. Stack the lettuce on the sauce on the bottom bun.

8. Stack the cheese on the lettuce.

9. Place one beef patty on the cheese.

10. The middle bun goes next with the sauce-coated side facing up.

11. Stack the other beef patty on the middle bun.

12. Finish the burger off with the top bun. You can microwave the burger for 10 to 15 seconds if you want to warm up the buns.

✳ Big Boy Club Sandwich

Serves 1 as an entree (can be doubled)

Menu Description: "Slices of turkey breast with bacon, tomato, lettuce and mayonnaise, stacked on toasted bread. Served with coleslaw."

When Bob Wian invented the first Big Boy double-decker hamburger in 1937, his restaurant business went through the roof. Soon a slew of imitators hit the market with their own giant-sized burgers: Bun Boy, Brawny Boy, Super Boy, Yumi Boy, Country Boy, Husky Boy, Hi-Boy, Beefy Boy, Lucky Boy, and many other "Boys" across the burger-crazed country.

By 1985 the Big Boy statues had become a common sight in front of hundreds of Bob's restaurants around the country. This was also the year the Marriott Corporation, which had purchased Bob's from a retiring Bob Wian in 1967, created a national ballot to decide whether the Big Boy character would stay or go. Thousands of voters elected to keep the tubby little tike, but his days were numbered. In 1992, Marriott chose to sell all of the Bob's Big Boys to an investment group. Those mostly West Coast Big Boys were later converted to Coco's or Carrow's restaurants, and there the Big Boy went bye-bye. The Elias Brothers, a Michigan-area franchiser for many years, purchased the Big Boy name from Marriott in 1987, and today is the sole Big Boy franchiser worldwide.

The Club Sandwich is one of Big Boy's signature sandwiches, and remains one of the most popular items on the menu since it was introduced in the mid-70s.

3 slices white or wheat bread	2 ounces deli-sliced turkey
1½ tablespoons mayonnaise	breast
1 lettuce leaf	2 slices tomato
1 slice Swiss cheese	3 slices bacon, cooked
(optional)	

1. Toast the slices of bread.
2. Spread the mayonnaise evenly on one face of each slice of toast.
3. Build the sandwich by first stacking the lettuce leaf on the may-

onnaise on one slice of toast. You will most likely have to cut or fold the lettuce so that it fits.

4. The Swiss cheese goes on next. This is an optional step since I've been served the original sandwich with the cheese, but the description of the sandwich and the photograph in the menu exclude it.

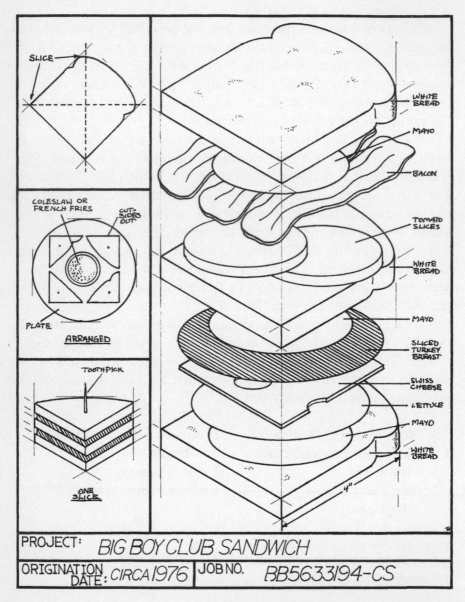

5. On the Swiss cheese, if you use it, stack the slices of turkey. Fold over the slices and arrange them neatly.
6. Stack a piece of toast, mayo side down, onto the turkey.
7. On top of the toast, arrange the tomato slices.
8. Lay the bacon, side by side, onto the tomatoes.
9. Top off the sandwich with the last piece of toast, mayo side down.
10. Slice the sandwich with two diagonal cuts from corner to corner, in an "x."
11. Push a toothpick down through the center of each triangular sandwich quarter. Spin each slice around 180 degrees so that the center of the sandwich is now pointed out. Serve with French fries or with coleslaw arranged in the center of the plate of sandwich pieces.

✳ California Pizza Kitchen Original BBQ Chicken Pizza

Serves 2 as an entree

Menu Description: *"Introduced in our first restaurant in 1985. With barbecued chicken, sliced red onion, cilantro, and smoked Gouda cheese."*

In 1985, attorneys Larry Flax and Rick Rosenfield traded in their private practice, which included defending mob bosses and union officials for a specialty pizza chain. These two "amateur chefs" say they were influenced by Wolfgang Puck, whose Spago restaurant in Los Angeles was the first to create pizza with unusual toppings. Now they have developed a niche somewhere between gourmet food and traditional Italian-style pizzas, creating what one magazine described as "designer pizza at off-the-rack prices." In addition to the pastas, soups, and salads on its nothing-over-ten-dollars menu, California Pizza Kitchen offers 25 unique pizza creations that reflect the current trends in dining. When Cajun food was in style, the Cajun chicken pizza was a top seller; today that item has been replaced with Southwestern pizza varieties.

As the menu explains, the Barbecued Chicken Pizza was one of the first pizzas served at California Pizza Kitchen. Ten years later it remains the top-selling pizza creation.

You can use this recipe to make your pizza with premade or packaged dough, but I highly recommend taking the time to make the dough yourself. You'll find that it's worth the extra work. This recipe took a lot of time to perfect, and if you prepare the dough one day ahead of time, the result should convince you never to use packaged dough again.

The Crust

⅓ cup plus 1 tablespoon warm water (105 degrees to 115 degrees F)

¾ teaspoon yeast
or

1 teaspoon sugar
1 cup bread flour
½ teaspoon salt
½ tablespoon olive oil

62

Commercial pizza dough	1 10-inch unbaked
or dough mix	commercial crust
or	

The Topping

1 boneless, skinless chicken breast half	½ cup grated Gouda cheese (smoked, if you can find it)
½ cup Bullseye Original barbecue sauce	½ cup sliced red onion
1½ teaspoons olive oil	2 teaspoons finely chopped fresh cilantro*
1 cup shredded mozzarella	

1. If you are making a homemade crust, start the dough one day before you plan to serve the pizza. In a small bowl or measuring cup dissolve the yeast and sugar in the warm water. Let it sit for 5 minutes until the surface of the mixture turns foamy. (If it doesn't foam, either the yeast was too old—i.e., dead—or the water was too hot—i.e., you killed it. Try again.) Sift together the flour and salt in a medium bowl. Make a depression in the flour and pour in the olive oil and yeast mixture. Use a fork to stir the liquid, gradually drawing in more flour as you stir, until all the ingredients are combined. When you can no longer stir with a fork, use your hands to form the dough into a ball. Knead the dough with the heels of your hands on a lightly floured surface for 10 minutes, or until the texture of the dough is smooth. Form the dough back into a ball, coat it lightly with oil, and place it into a clean bowl covered with plastic wrap. Keep the bowl in a warm place for about 2 hours to allow the dough to double in size. Punch down the dough and put it back into the covered bowl and into your refrigerator overnight. Take the dough from the refrigerator 1 to 2 hours before you plan to build the pizza so that the dough can warm up to room temperature.

   If you are using a commercial dough or dough mix, follow the instructions on the package to prepare it. You may have to set some of the dough aside to make a smaller, 10-inch crust.

*Found in the produce section near the parsley. Also known as fresh coriander or Chinese parsley.

63

2. Cut the chicken breast into bite-size cubes and marinate it in ¼ cup of the barbecue sauce in the refrigerator for at least 2 hours.
3. When the chicken has marinated, preheat the oven to 500 degrees F. Heat a small frying pan on your stove with about 1½ teaspoons of olive oil in it. Sauté the chicken in the pan for about 3 to 4 minutes or until done.

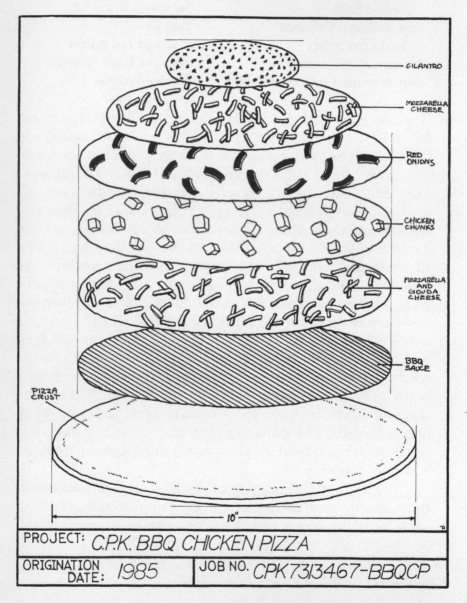

CILANTRO

MOZZARELLA CHEESE

RED ONIONS

CHICKEN CHUNKS

MOZZARELLA AND GOUDA CHEESE

BBQ SAUCE

PIZZA CRUST

|← 10" →|

PROJECT: *C.P.K. BBQ CHICKEN PIZZA*

ORIGINATION DATE: *1985*   JOB NO. *CPK 7313467-BBQCP*

4. Form the dough into a ball and roll out on a floured surface until very thin and 10 inches in diameter. Put your pizza crust onto a baking sheet or pizza pan, and spread the remaining ¼ cup of barbecue sauce evenly over the pizza crust.
5. Sprinkle ½ cup of the mozzarella and all of the Gouda cheese over the sauce.
6. Add the chicken next.
7. The red onion goes next.
8. Sprinkle the remaining ½ cup mozzarella around the center of the pizza.
9. Cilantro goes on top of the mozzarella.
10. Bake the pizza for 10 to 12 minutes or until the crust is light brown.
11. When the pizza is done, remove it from the oven and make 4 even cuts across the pie. This will give you 8 slices.

✳ California Pizza Kitchen Thai Chicken Pizza

Serves 2 as an entree

Menu Description: *"With pieces of chicken marinated in a spicy peanut-ginger and sesame sauce, green onions, bean sprouts, julienne carrots, cilantro and roasted peanuts."*

After the first California Pizza Kitchen opened in Beverly Hills in 1985 success came quickly: there are currently 78 restaurants in 18 states. In 1992, huge food conglomerate PepsiCo paid over $70 million for a 70 percent share of the company—just eight years after Larry and Rick started the company. As for those two, well, they pocketed $18 million apiece, or around 70 times their initial investment in 1985.

Thai Chicken Pizza is one of the oldest varieties of pizza still on the menu, and remains a favorite. If you prefer, you can make this pizza with a store-bought package dough or dough mix, but I recommend making the crust yourself. If you decide to do that, make it one day ahead of time so that it can rise slowly in the refrigerator.

The Crust

⅓ cup plus 1 tablespoon warm water (105 degrees to 115 degrees F)
¾ teaspoon yeast
1 teaspoon granulated sugar
1 cup bread flour
½ teaspoon salt

½ tablespoon olive oil
or
Commercial pizza dough or dough mix
or
1 10-inch unbaked commercial crust

Peanut Sauce

¼ cup creamy peanut butter
2 tablespoons teriyaki sauce (or marinade)
2 tablespoons hoisin

1 tablespoon brown sugar
2 tablespoons water
2 teaspoons sesame oil
1 teaspoon soy sauce
1½ teaspoons minced onion

66

| 1 clove garlic, minced | 1 teaspoon minced |
| ½ teaspoon crushed red pepper flakes | gingerroot |

Toppings

1 boneless, skinless chicken breast half	½ carrot, julienned or grated (¼ cup)
1½ teaspoons olive oil	2 teaspoons minced cilantro*
1¼ cups grated mozzarella	
1 to 2 green onions	1 tablespoon chopped peanuts
½ cup bean sprouts	

1. Prepare the crust following the directions from step 1 on page 63.
2. Mix together the ingredients for the peanut sauce in a small bowl. Pour this mixture into a food processor or blender and blend for about 15 seconds or until the garlic, onion, and ginger are reduced to small particles. Pour this mixture into a small pan over medium heat and bring it to a boil. Cook for 1 minute. Don't cook too long or the sauce will become lumpy. (You may, instead, use a microwave for this step. Pour the mixture into a small microwavable bowl and heat for 1 to 2 minutes.) The peanut sauce should be darker now.
3. Slice the chicken into bite-size chunks.
4. Pour one-third of the peanut sauce over the chicken in a sealed container in the refrigerator and marinate for at least 2 hours. I like to use a small resealable plastic bag for this. The chicken gets very well coated this way.
5. Heat 1 teaspoon of oil in a small pan over medium/high heat.
6. Cook the marinated chicken for 3 to 4 minutes in the pan.
7. Roll out your pizza crust and place on the baking sheet or pizza pan as in step 4, page 65. Preheat the oven to 475 degrees F.
8. Spread a thin coating of the remaining peanut sauce (the stuff you *didn't* marinate the chicken in) on the pizza crust. You may have sauce left over.
9. Sprinkle 1 cup of the grated mozzarella over the peanut sauce.

*Cilantro is found in the produce section of your supermarket, usually near the parsley.

10. Slice the green onion lengthwise into thin strips (julienne), then cut across the strips, slicing the onion into 2-inch matchstick strips. Spread the onions over the cheese.
11. Arrange the chicken on the pizza.
12. Next go the sprouts and the julienned carrots.

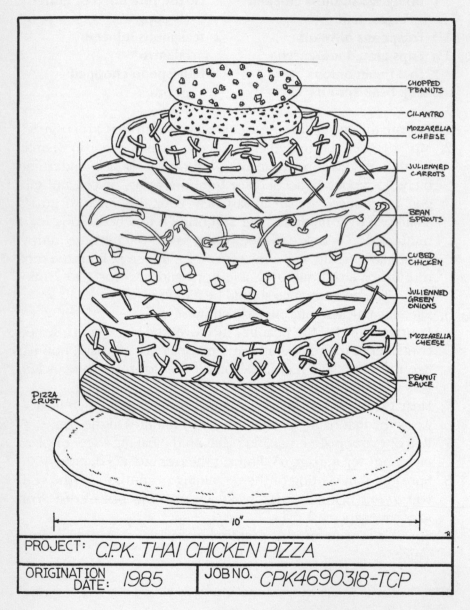

CHOPPED PEANUTS

CILANTRO

MOZZARELLA CHEESE

JULIENNED CARROTS

BEAN SPROUTS

CUBED CHICKEN

JULIENNED GREEN ONIONS

MOZZARELLA CHEESE

PEANUT SAUCE

PIZZA CRUST

10"

PROJECT: C.P.K. THAI CHICKEN PIZZA

ORIGINATION DATE: 1985

JOB NO. CPK4690318-TCP

68

13. Sprinkle what's left of the mozzarella (¼ cup) just over the center area of the pizza.
14. Sprinkle the cilantro over the mozzarella, then the chopped nuts on top.
15. Bake the pizza for 10 to 12 minutes or until the crust turns light brown.
16. After removing the pizza from the oven, cut across it 4 times to make 8 slices.

✳ California Pizza Kitchen Southwestern Burrito Pizza

Serves 2 as an entree

Menu Description: "With grilled chicken breast marinated in lime and herbs, Southwestern black beans, fire-roasted mild chilies, sweet white onions and Cheddar cheese. Served with green tomatillo salsa and sour cream."

California Pizza Kitchen uses imported Italian wood-fired ovens to bake the specialty pizzas. These ovens reach temperatures over 800 degrees F, allowing the pizzas to cook in just three minutes. This technique keeps ingredients from drying out so that the pizzas don't require as much cheese as in traditional recipes.

Unfortunately, most of us don't have wood-burning pizza ovens in our kitchens so I have designed these recipes to work in a conventional oven with a minimum of cheese. If you have a pizza stone, use it. If you have a hard time finding tomatillos (they look like small green tomatoes with a thin papery skin and are found in the produce section), you can use canned green salsa. Look for fresh cilantro in the produce section.

You have the option of using a store-bought crust or instant pizza dough, but I can't say enough about making the dough yourself from the recipe here. You just have to plan ahead, making the dough one day before you plan to bake the pizza. This way the dough will get to rest and will rise slowly in the refrigerator—a great technique the pros use.

The Crust

⅓ cup plus 1 tablespoon warm water (105 degrees to 115 degrees F)
¾ teaspoon yeast
1 teaspoon sugar
1 cup bread flour
½ teaspoon salt

½ tablespoon olive oil
or
1 10-inch unbaked commercial crust
or
Commercial pizza dough or dough mix

70

Marinated Chicken

1 tablespoon fresh lime juice
1 tablespoon plus 1 teaspoon
    olive oil
1 tablespoon soy sauce
2 cloves garlic, pressed
2 teaspoons chopped fresh
    cilantro
1 teaspoon salt
½ teaspoon crushed red
    pepper flakes
1 skinless, boneless chicken
    breast half

¾ cup canned refried black
    beans
1 tablespoon water
¼ teaspoon cayenne pepper
¼ cup sliced white onion
1 whole canned mild green
    chili
½ cup shredded Monterey
    Jack cheese
1 cup shredded Cheddar
    cheese

Tomatillo Salsa (optional)

¾ cup chopped tomatillos
    (about 4)
3 whole canned mild green
    chilies (4-ounce can)

¼ fresh jalapeño
2 tablespoons chopped
    onion
Dash salt

On the Side

Sour cream

1. Prepare the crust following directions from step 1 on page 63.
2. Make the marinade by combining the lime juice, 1 tablespoon olive oil, soy sauce, garlic, cilantro, salt, and pepper flakes in a blender or in a small bowl with an electric mixer for only 5 seconds or so, just until the ingredients are well combined.
3. Cut the chicken into bite-size cubes, then marinate the chicken breast in the lime mixture for at least 2 hours.
4. When the chicken has marinated, heat up a small skillet with the remaining 1 teaspoon of olive oil over high heat. Cook the chicken in the pan for 2 to 4 minutes or until it is cooked through.
5. Mix the black beans with the water and cayenne pepper.
6. Roll out the pizza crust and place it on the baking sheet or pizza pan as in step 4, page 65. Preheat the oven to 475 degrees F.

7. Spread the black bean mixture evenly over the crust.
8. Now arrange the chicken evenly over the black beans.
9. Spread the onions over the chicken.
10. Take the chili pepper and carefully slice it in half, crossways. Then slice the two halves into very thin strips. Sprinkle the chili over the onions.

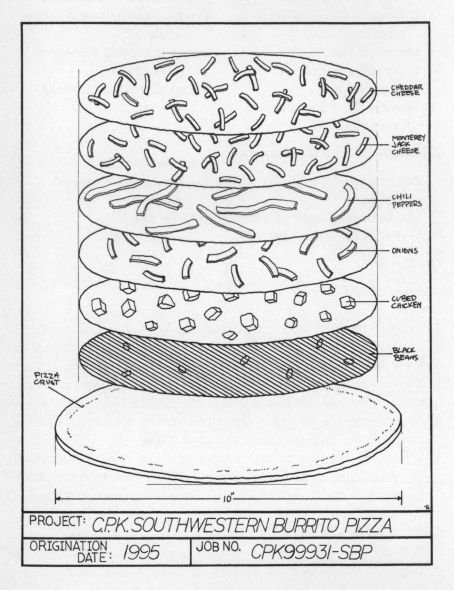

CHEDDAR CHEESE

MONTEREY JACK CHEESE

CHILI PEPPERS

ONIONS

CUBED CHICKEN

BLACK BEANS

PIZZA CRUST

|←————————— 10" —————————→|

PROJECT: *C.P.K. SOUTHWESTERN BURRITO PIZZA*

ORIGINATION DATE: *1995*   JOB NO. *CPK99931-SBP*

11. Spread the Monterey Jack over the pizza.
12. Top it off with the Cheddar.
13. Cook the pizza for 12 to 15 minutes or until the crust begins to turn brown.
14. While the pizza cooks, combine all the ingredients for the tomatillo salsa in a food processor or blender. Run on low speed for about 15 seconds.
15. When the pizza is done, remove it from the oven and immediately make 4 even cuts through the middle, creating 8 slices of pizza. Serve with tomatillo sauce and sour cream on the side.

✳ The Cheesecake Factory Bruschetta

Serves 2 as an appetizer

Menu Description: "Grilled Bread Topped with Fresh Chopped Tomato, Red Onion, Garlic, Basil and Olive Oil."

In 1972, Oscar and Evelyn Overton moved from Detroit to Los Angeles to build a wholesale bakery that would sell cheesecakes and other high-quality desserts to local restaurants. Business was a booming success, but some restaurants balked at the high prices the bakery was charging for its desserts. So in 1978 the couple's son David decided to open a restaurant of his own—the first Cheesecake Factory restaurant—in posh Beverly Hills. The restaurant was an immediate success and soon David started a moderate expansion of the concept. Sure, the current total of 20 restaurants doesn't seem like a lot, but this handful of stores earns the chain more than $100 million in business each year. That's more than some chains with four times the number of outlets rake in.

Bruschetta is one of the top-selling appetizers at the restaurant chain. Bruschetta is toasted bread flavored with garlic and olive oil, broiled until crispy, and then arranged around a pile of tomato-basil salad in vinaigrette. This salad is scooped onto the bruschetta, like a dip, and then you open wide. This version makes five slices just like the dish served at the restaurant, but the recipe can be easily doubled.

1½ cups chopped Roma
    plum tomatoes
    (6 to 8 tomatoes)
2 tablespoons diced red
    onion
1 large clove garlic, minced
2 tablespoons chopped fresh
    basil (4 to 6 small leaves)
2 tablespoons olive oil

½ teaspoon red wine vinegar
¼ teaspoon salt
Dash ground black
    pepper
½ loaf French baguette or
    crusty Italian bread
    (5 to 7 slices)
¼ teaspoon garlic salt
2 to 3 sprigs Italian parsley

1. Combine the tomatoes, red onion, garlic, and basil in a medium bowl.
2. Add ½ tablespoon of oil, vinegar, salt, and pepper and mix well. Cover the bowl and let it sit in the refrigerator for at least 1 hour.

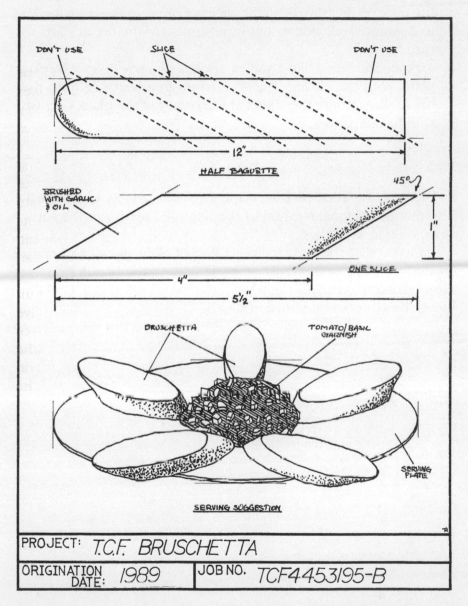

DON'T USE   SLICE   DON'T USE

12"

HALF BAGUETTE

BRUSHED WITH GARLIC & OIL

45°

1"

4"

5½"

ONE SLICE

BRUSCHETTA   TOMATO/BASIL GARNISH

SERVING PLATE

SERVING SUGGESTION

PROJECT: T.C.F. BRUSCHETTA

ORIGINATION DATE: 1989   JOB NO. TCF4453195-B

3. When you are ready to serve the dish, preheat your broiler and slice the baguette in 1-inch slices on a 45-degree angle to make 5 slices of bread.
4. Combine the remaining 1½ tablespoons of oil with the garlic salt.
5. Brush the entire surface of each slice of bread (both sides) with the olive oil mixture. Broil the slices of bread in the oven for 1½ to 2 minutes per side or until the surface of the bread starts to turn brown.
6. Arrange the bread like a star or spokes of a wheel on a serving plate. Pour the chilled tomato mixture in a neat pile onto the bread slices where they meet at the center of the plate. Garnish with Italian parsley.

Tidbits

There is a variation on this recipe if your bread has a hard crust. The more traditional method of rubbing the bread with the garlic clove is done as follows:

After you slice the bread, slice a clove of garlic in half and rub it around the edge of the crust on both sides of the bread. Rub the olive oil on the bread and lightly salt each slice, if you like. Grill the bread the same way as above in step 5.

✳ The Cheesecake Factory
Avocado Eggrolls

Serves 1 or 2 as an appetizer

Menu Description: "Chunks of Fresh Avocado, Sun-Dried Tomato, Red Onion and Cilantro Deep Fried in a Crisp Chinese Wrapper."

In 1995, Forbes Magazine named the Cheesecake Factory in its list of the 200 best small companies in America. At 20 stores now, the Cheesecake Factory plans to grow at a modest rate of about 5 new restaurants per year, and still does not franchise.

Here's something different that I think you'll really like. The Avocado Eggrolls are one of the most popular appetizers on the menu at the Cheesecake Factory, and it's not hard to see why. The combination of hot avocado, sun-dried tomatoes, and the cilantro-tamarind sauce is one of the most unique and tasty flavors I've enjoyed at any of the restaurant chains. The trickiest part might be finding the tamarind pulp at your market. It's a brown, sticky pulp that looks sort of like puréed prunes, and can be found in the spice section or near the ethnic foods—or try a Middle Eastern market. The pulp often contains the large seeds of the fruit, so be sure to remove them before measuring. If you can't find the tamarind, you can get by substituting smashed raisins or prunes.

Eggrolls

1 large avocado	½ teaspoon chopped fresh
2 tablespoons chopped	cilantro
sun-dried tomatoes	Pinch salt
(bottled in oil)	3 eggroll wrappers
1 tablespoon minced red	1 egg, beaten
onion	Vegetable oil for frying

Dipping Sauce

¼ cup chopped cashews
⅔ cup chopped fresh cilantro
2 cloves garlic, quartered
2 green onions, chopped
1 tablespoon sugar
1 teaspoon ground black
　　pepper

1 teaspoon cumin
4 teaspoons white vinegar
1 teaspoon balsamic vinegar
½ teaspoon tamarind pulp
½ cup honey
Pinch ground saffron
¼ cup olive oil

1. After you peel the avocado and remove the pit, dice it into bite-size pieces.
2. In a small bowl, gently combine the avocado with the tomatoes, red onion, ½ teaspoon cilantro, and a pinch of salt. Be careful not to smash the avocado.
3. Prepare the eggrolls by spooning ⅓ of the filling into an eggroll wrapper. With the wrapper positioned so that one corner is pointing toward you, place the filling about 1 inch from the bottom corner and 1 inch from each side. Roll the bottom corner up over the filling, then roll the filling up to about the middle of the wrapper. Brush the remaining corners and edges of the wrapper with the beaten egg. Fold the left and right corners over the filling and "glue" the corners to the wrapper. Finish by rolling the wrapper and filling up over the top corner. Press on the wrapper to ensure it is sealed. Repeat these steps with the remaining two eggrolls and keep them covered in the refrigerator while you make the dipping sauce.
4. Prepare the sauce by combining the cashews, cilantro, garlic, green onions, sugar, black pepper, and cumin in a food processor or blender. Blend with short bursts until the mixture is well blended, and the cashews and garlic have been chopped into pieces about half the size of a grain of rice.
5. Combine the vinegars, honey, tamarind, and saffron in a small bowl. Heat the mixture for about 1 minute in a microwave, then stir until the tamarind pulp dissolves completely.
6. Pour the tamarind mixture into the blender or food processor with the cashew mixture and mix with short bursts until well combined (about 20 seconds).
7. Pour the blended sauce into a small bowl. Add the oil and stir by hand. Cover and refrigerate the sauce for at least 30 minutes before serving.

8. Heat oil in a deep fryer or a deep pan over medium heat. You want the oil to be deep enough to cover the eggrolls.
9. When the oil is hot, fry the eggrolls for 3 to 4 minutes or until golden brown. Drain on paper towels.
10. When the eggrolls can be safely touched, slice once diagonally across the middle of each one and serve them arranged around a sauce dish filled with the dipping sauce.

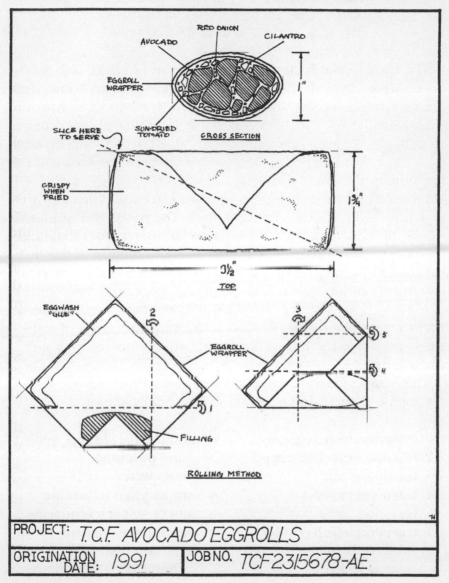

PROJECT: T.C.F AVOCADO EGGROLLS

ORIGINATION DATE: 1991   JOB NO. TCF2315678-AE

✳ The Cheesecake Factory Cajun Jambalaya Pasta

Serves 2 as a large entree

Menu Description: "Our most popular dish! Shrimp and Chicken Sautéed with Onions, Peppers and Tomatoes in a Very Spicy Cajun Sauce. All on top of Fresh Fettuccine."

The Cheesecake Factory's founder, David Overton, says it was his unfamiliarity with the restaurant business that contributed to the company's success. In an interview with *Nation's Restaurant News* David says, "We did not know anything about running restaurants. We just knew that people valued fresh foods. In some ways our naiveté helped us because we didn't know what you are not supposed to do."

I think we all know it helps to serve good food and that's an area in which the Cheesecake Factory excels. The pastas and salads top the list of big sellers, but it's the Cajun Jambalaya Pasta that holds the pole position, according to the menu description of this dish. Jambalaya is a spicy Creole dish that usually combines a variety of ingredients including tomatoes, onions, peppers, and some type of meat with rice. Rather than the traditional rice, the Cheesecake Factory has designed its version to include two types of fettuccine—an attractive mix of standard white noodles and green spinach-flavored noodles.

This recipe makes 2 huge portions, like those served in the restaurant. It's actually enough food for a family of four.

½ teaspoon white pepper
½ teaspoon cayenne pepper
1½ teaspoons salt
½ teaspoon paprika
¼ teaspoon garlic powder
¼ teaspoon onion powder
2 skinless, boneless chicken breast halves

½ pound large shrimp, peeled and deveined
5 quarts water
6 ounces plain fettuccine
6 ounces spinach fettuccine
2 tablespoons olive oil
2 medium tomatoes, chopped

1 small green bell pepper, sliced	1½ cups chicken stock
1 small red bell pepper, sliced	1 tablespoon arrowroot or cornstarch
1 small yellow bell pepper, sliced	2 tablespoons white wine
1 small white onion, sliced	2 teaspoons chopped fresh parsley

1. Make a Cajun seasoning blend by combining the white pepper, cayenne pepper, salt, paprika, garlic powder, and onion powder in a small bowl.
2. Cut the chicken breasts into bite-size pieces. Use about one-third of the seasoning blend to coat the chicken pieces.
3. In another bowl, sprinkle another one-third of the spice blend over the shrimp.
4. Start your pasta cooking by bringing 5 quarts of water to a boil over high heat. Add both fettuccines to the hot water, reduce the heat to medium, and simmer for 12 to 14 minutes or until the pasta is tender.
5. While the fettuccine cooks, heat 1 tablespoon of the olive oil in a large frying pan or skillet over high heat. When the oil is hot, sauté the chicken in the pan for about 2 minutes per side or until the surface of the chicken starts to turn brown.
6. Add the shrimp to the pan with the chicken and cook for another 2 minutes, stirring occasionally to keep the shrimp from sticking. When the chicken and shrimp have been seared, pour the contents of the pan onto a plate or into a bowl. Do not rinse the pan!
7. Put the pan back over the high heat and add the remaining tablespoon of oil to the pan. Add the tomatoes, peppers, and onion to the oil. Sprinkle the veggies with the remaining spice blend and sauté for about 10 minutes or until the vegetables begin to turn dark brown or black.
8. Add the chicken and shrimp to the vegetables and pour ¾ cup of the chicken stock in the pan. Cook over high heat until the stock has been reduced to just about nothing. Add the remaining ¾ cup of the stock to the pan. The liquid should become dark as it deglazes the pan of the dark film left by the spices and cooking food. Stir constantly, scraping the blackened stuff on

the bottom of the pan. Reduce the broth a bit more, then turn the heat down to low.

9. Combine the arrowroot with the wine in a small bowl. Stir until it is dissolved. Add this to the pan and simmer over low heat until the sauce thickens slightly.

10. When the fettuccine is done, drain it and spoon half onto a plate. Spoon half of the jambalaya over the fettuccine. Sprinkle half of the parsley over the top. Repeat for the second serving.

Tidbits

You may also be able to find fettuccine that comes in a 12-ounce box with a combination of plain and spinach noodles. One brand is Ronzoni. This variety is perfect for this recipe, and you won't have any leftover noodles in opened boxes.

✳ The Cheesecake Factory
Pumpkin Cheesecake

Serves 8

While most restaurant chains attempt to keep their menus simple so as to not tax the kitchen, the Cheesecake Factory's menu contains more than 200 items. Perhaps it's the time spent reading the 17-page menu that leads to the one- and two-hour waits for a table that customers not only expect, but cheerfully endure for lunch or dinner, or just for a taste of the delicious Pumpkin Cheesecake or any of the other 40 cheesecake selections.

Use an 8-inch springform pan for this recipe. If you don't have one, you should get one. They're indispensable for thick, gourmet cheesecake and several other scrumptious desserts. If you don't want to use a springform pan, this recipe will also work with two 9-inch pie plates. You'll just end up with two smaller cheesecakes.

1½ cups graham cracker
    crumbs
5 tablespoons butter, melted
1 cup plus 1 tablespoon
    sugar
3 8-ounce packages cream
    cheese, softened

1 teaspoon vanilla
1 cup canned pumpkin
3 eggs
½ teaspoon cinnamon
¼ teaspoon nutmeg
¼ teaspoon allspice
Whipped cream

1. Preheat the oven to 350 degrees F.
2. Make the crust by combining the graham cracker crumbs with the melted butter and 1 tablespoon sugar in a medium bowl. Stir well enough to coat all of the crumbs with the butter, but not so much as to turn the mixture into paste. Keep it crumbly.
3. Press the crumbs onto the bottom and about two-thirds of the way up the sides of the springform pan. You don't want the crust to form all of the way up the back of each slice of cheesecake. Bake the crust for 5 minutes, then set it aside until you are ready to fill it.

4. In a large mixing bowl combine the cream cheese, 1 cup sugar, and vanilla. Mix with an electric mixer until smooth.
5. Add the pumpkin, eggs, cinnamon, nutmeg, and allspice and continue to beat until smooth and creamy.

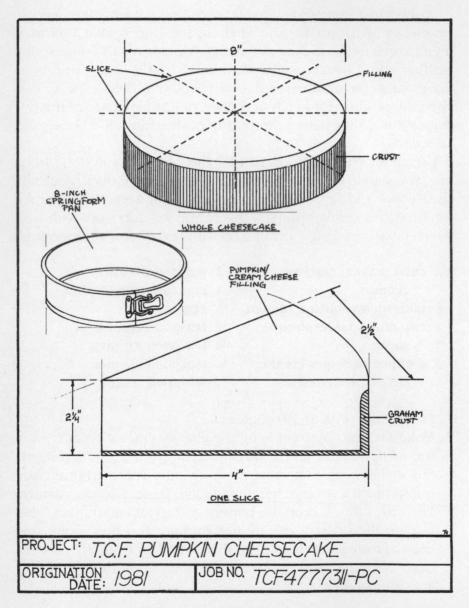

SLICE

FILLING

8"

CRUST

8-INCH
SPRINGFORM
PAN

WHOLE CHEESECAKE

PUMPKIN/
CREAM CHEESE
FILLING

2½"

2¼"

GRAHAM
CRUST

4"

ONE SLICE

PROJECT: T.C.F. PUMPKIN CHEESECAKE

ORIGINATION DATE: 1981

JOB NO. TCF4777311-PC

84

6. Pour the filling into the pan. Bake for 60 to 70 minutes. The top will turn a bit darker at this point. Remove from the oven and allow the cheesecake to cool.

7. When the cheesecake has come to room temperature, put it into the refrigerator. When the cheesecake has chilled, remove the pan sides and cut the cake into 8 equal pieces. Serve with a generous portion of whipped cream on top.

✳ The Cheesecake Factory Key Lime Cheesecake

Serves 8

Just 15 minutes after the very first Cheesecake Factory opened in Beverly Hills back in 1978, the lines began forming. Here's their cheesecake twist on the delicious Key lime pie. Since Key limes and Key lime juice can be hard to find, this recipe uses standard lime juice, which can be purchased bottled or squeezed fresh. If you can find Key lime juice, bear in mind that Key limes are more tart, and use only half as much juice. This recipe also requires a springform pan. If you don't have one, you can use two 9-inch pie pans and make two smaller cheesecakes.

1¾ cups graham cracker
 crumbs
5 tablespoons butter, melted
1 cup plus 1 tablespoon
 sugar
3 8-ounce packages cream
 cheese, softened

1 teaspoon vanilla
½ cup fresh lime juice
 (about 5 limes)
3 eggs
 Whipped cream

1. Preheat the oven to 350 degrees F. Make the crust by combining the graham cracker crumbs with the butter and 1 tablespoon sugar in a medium bowl. Stir well enough to coat all of the crumbs with the butter. Keep it crumbly.
2. Press the crumbs onto the bottom and about one half of the way up the sides of an 8-inch springform pan. You don't want the crust to form all the way up the back of each slice of cheesecake. Bake the crust for 5 minutes, then set it aside until you are ready to fill it.
3. In a large mixing bowl combine the cream cheese, 1 cup sugar, and vanilla. Mix with an electric mixer until smooth.
4. Add the lime juice and eggs and continue to beat until smooth and creamy.
5. Pour the filling into the pan. Bake for 60 to 70 minutes. If the

top of the cheesecake is turning light brown, it's done. Remove from the oven and allow it to cool.

6. When the cheesecake has come to room temperature, put it into the refrigerator. When the cheesecake has chilled, remove the pan sides and cut the cake into 8 equal pieces. Serve with a generous dollop of whipped cream on top.

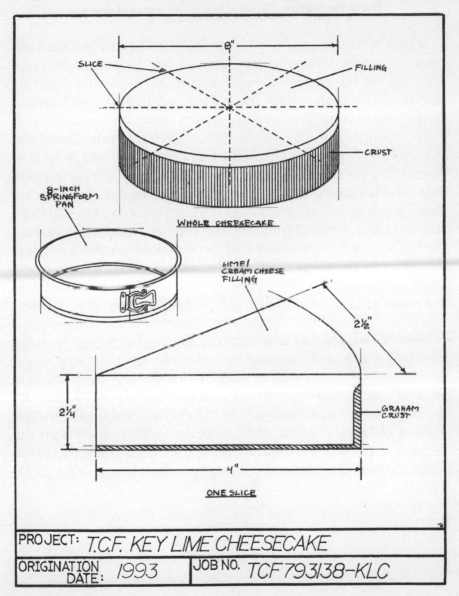

SLICE   8"   FILLING

CRUST

8-INCH
SPRINGFORM
PAN

WHOLE CHEESECAKE

LIME/
CREAM CHEESE
FILLING

2½"

2¼"

GRAHAM
CRUST

4"

ONE SLICE

PROJECT: T.C.F. KEY LIME CHEESECAKE

ORIGINATION DATE: 1993   JOB NO. TCF 793138-KLC

87

✳ Chi-Chi's Nachos Grande

Serves 2 to 4 as an appetizer

Menu Description: *"Seasoned beef, refried beans and cheese."*

Marno McDermott was a successful Minneapolis restaurateur, opening a chain of Mexican restaurants in the seventies called Zapata's against the advice of skeptics who said he would never be able to sell Mexican food to the large population of Scandinavians in the area. Marno proved them wrong then, and once again in 1976, when he partnered with Max McGee, a former Green Bay Packer football player, to open the first Chi-Chi's in Richfield, Minnesota. The restaurant was built inside a deserted Kroger grocery store and became instantly famous for the intensely flavored and larger-than-usual portions of food. To keep volume high, Chi-Chi's designed a custom computer-driven system that clocks every aspect of service from the time each server enters an order to when the order is placed in front of customers. Special attention was given to the design of the menus items as well, with each dish taking no more than nine minutes to prepare, even during the rush hours.

Since you're starting from scratch, this appetizer will probably take longer than nine minutes to make, but not by much. At the restaurant you can order the Nachos Grande with beef, chicken, seafood, or a combination; here I've described methods to recreate the beef and chicken versions. You can choose to make the nachos from store-bought tortilla chips or make them yourself with the recipe in "Tidbits." Personally I think the fresh, home-fried type tastes the best. If you're up for the task, amigos, I say give it a go.

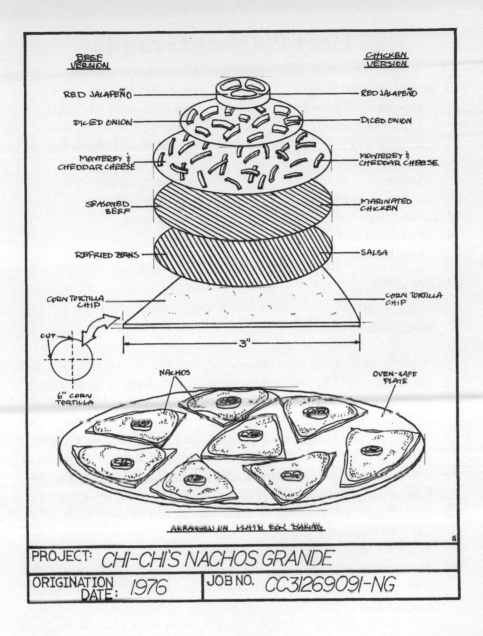

PROJECT: *CHI-CHI'S NACHOS GRANDE*

ORIGINATION DATE: 1976

JOB NO. CC3l269091-NG

89

✳ Beef Nachos Grande

½ pound ground beef
1 teaspoon chili powder
   (Spanish blend)
½ teaspoon salt
½ teaspoon dried minced
   onion
⅛ teaspoon paprika
2 tablespoons water
8 "restaurant-style" corn
   tortilla chips

½ cup refried beans
1½ cups shredded Cheddar
   cheese
½ cup shredded Monterey
   Jack cheese
¼ cup diced onion
1 large red jalapeño
   (or green)

On the Side

Sour cream   Salsa
Guacamole

1. Preheat the oven to 375 degrees F.
2. Brown the ground beef in a skillet over medium heat. Use a spatula or fork to crumble the beef into small pieces as it cooks. When you no longer see pink in the meat, drain off the fat.
3. To the meat, add the chili powder, salt, dried onion, paprika, and water. Simmer over medium/low heat for 10 minutes.
4. If you are going to prepare your own tortilla chips, do that following the instructions in "Tidbits" while the meat is simmering.
5. Heat the refried beans in a small saucepan over low heat or in the microwave for about 2 minutes.
6. Mix the two cheeses together in a small bowl.
7. Arrange the tortilla chips on a baking sheet or an oven-safe ceramic plate. Spread about a tablespoon of refried beans on each chip.
8. Sprinkle a couple of tablespoons of spiced beef onto the beans on each chip. Press down on the beef to make a flat surface for the cheese.
9. Carefully pile a small handful of cheese on each chip.
10. Sprinkle a pinch of the diced onion over the cheese.
11. Place a slice of jalapeño on top of the onion.

12. Bake the chips for 8 to 10 minutes or until the cheese has melted. Serve with your choice of sour cream, guacamole, and salsa on the side.

✳ Chicken Nachos Grande

2 tablespoons lime juice
¼ cup water
1 tablespoon vegetable oil
¼ teaspoon liquid smoke
2 teaspoons vinegar
1 clove garlic, pressed
   Salt
   Pepper
1 boneless, skinless chicken
   breast

1 cup salsa
1½ cups shredded Cheddar
   cheese
½ cup shredded Monterey
   Jack cheese
¼ cup diced onion
1 large red jalapeño pepper
   (or green)

1. Combine the lime juice, water, oil, liquid smoke, vinegar, and garlic. Add a little salt and pepper and marinate the chicken in the mixture for at least 2 hours.
2. Grill the chicken on your preheated barbecue or stovetop grill or griddle for 4 to 5 minutes per side or until done. Dice the chicken. Preheat the oven to 375 degrees F.
3. Instead of refried beans as in the previous recipe, spread 1 tablespoon of salsa on each of the eight chips. Sprinkle some chicken over the top and build the rest of the nacho the same way as the beef version: Cheeses, onion, then a jalapeño slice.
4. Bake for 8 to 10 minutes. Serve with sour cream, guacamole, and additional salsa on the side.

Tidbits

If you want to make your own tasty tortilla chips, buy some 6-inch corn tortillas and cut two of them twice—like a small pizza—into 4 equal triangular pieces (making a total of 8 slices).

91

Drop the tortilla slices 4 at a time into a frying pan filled with about ½ inch of oil that has preheated over medium heat. Chips should bubble rapidly and will only need to fry 30 to 45 seconds per side. They should become a bit more golden in color, and very crispy. Drain the chips on a rack or on some paper towels. Salt to taste.

✳ Chi-Chi's Sweet Corn Cake

Serves 8 to 10 as a side dish

Chi-Chi's cofounder Max McDermott named his restaurant chain after his wife Chi Chi. He claims the name is quite memorable as it translates in Spanish into something a lot like "hooters" in English. The Minneapolis Star quoted McDermott in 1977 shortly after the first Chi-Chi's opened in Richfield, Minneapolis, "English-speaking patrons remember it because it's catchy. And the Spanish-speaking customers are amused. Either way it doesn't hurt business."

One of the side dishes included with several of the entrees at Chi-Chi's is the Sweet Corn Cake. It's sort of like cornbread but much softer and sweeter, almost like corn pudding. You'll find it goes well with just about any Mexican dish. The recipe incorporates a *bain marie* or water bath—a technique of baking used commonly for custards and mousses to keep them from cracking or curdling. This is done by simply placing the covered baking pan of batter into another larger pan filled with a little hot water before baking.

½ cup (1 stick) butter, softened	¼ cup cornmeal
⅓ cup masa harina*	⅓ cup sugar
¼ cup water	2 tablespoons heavy cream
1½ cups frozen corn, thawed	¼ teaspoon salt
	½ teaspoon baking powder

1. Preheat the oven to 375 degrees F.
2. Blend the butter in a medium bowl with an electric mixer until creamy. Add the masa harina and water to the butter and beat until well combined.
3. Put the defrosted corn into a blender or food processor and, with short pulses, coarsely chop the corn on low speed. You

*A Mexican corn flour used to make tortillas. It is usually found in Latin-American groceries and in the supermarket next to the flour.

want to leave several whole kernels of corn. Stir the chopped corn into the butter and masa harina mixture. Add the cornmeal to the mixture. Combine.

4. In another medium bowl, mix together the sugar, cream, salt, and baking powder. When the ingredients are well blended, pour the mixture into the other bowl and stir everything together by hand.

5. Pour the corn batter into an ungreased 8×8-inch baking pan. Smooth the surface of the batter with a spatula. Cover the pan with aluminum foil. Place this pan into a 13×9-inch pan filled one-third of the way up with hot water. Bake for 50 to 60 minutes or until the corn cake is cooked through.

6. When the corn cake is done, remove the small pan from the larger pan and let it sit for at least 10 minutes. To serve, scoop out each portion with an ice cream scoop or rounded spoon.

✳ Chi-Chi's Twice Grilled Barbecue Burrito

Serves 2 as an entree

Menu Description: "Grilled steak or chicken wrapped in a flour tortilla with cheese and sautéed vegetables. Then the burrito is basted with spicy barbecue sauce and grilled again. Served with Spanish rice and sweet corn cake."

.This dish bursts with the Southwestern flavors that have become so popular lately. Southwestern dishes like fajitas and specialty burritos are the latest rage in the restaurant industry, and now more chains than ever are creating their own spicy, Southwestern-style goodies.

I think you'll really enjoy this one. Chi-Chi's has taken fajita-style grilled beef, rolled it up like a burrito, grilled it again, and then smothered it with smoky barbecue sauce. The dish has quickly become a favorite menu item at Chi-Chi's and a favorite for people tiring of the same old Mexican food. Fire up the grill and give this zesty recipe a try.

Marinade

⅓ cup water	½ teaspoon liquid smoke
¼ cup lime juice	½ teaspoon chili powder
1 large clove garlic, pressed or grated	½ teaspoon cayenne pepper
2 tablespoons vegetable oil	1 teaspoon salt
2 teaspoons vinegar	¼ teaspoon pepper
2 teaspoons soy sauce	Dash of onion powder

1 pound sirloin steak	2 tablespoons vegetable oil
1 red bell pepper, sliced	2 10-inch flour tortillas
1 green bell pepper, sliced	3 tablespoons Bullseye original barbecue sauce
1 Spanish onion, sliced	

1. Combine all of the ingredients for the marinade in a small bowl. Set aside ¼ cup of the marinade. Store it in a sealed container

95

in the fridge until you need it. Marinate the steak in the refrigerator with the remaining marinade for several hours. Overnight is best. Be sure the steak isn't too thick. If it's more than ½ inch thick, slice it thinner.

2. Grill the steak on a hot barbecue or preheated stovetop grill for 4 to 5 minutes per side or until done. Cook less for a rarer steak, longer if you want it well done.

3. While the steak grills, sauté the peppers and onion in 1 tablespoon of vegetable oil over high heat. When the vegetables are tender, add the ¼ cup of marinade you set aside. Continue sautéing the vegetables until they brown.

4. When the steak is done, slice it into long strips that are no more than ½ inch thick and ½ inch wide. Keep the grill on.

5. Lay the tortillas in a hot pan over low heat to make them warm and pliable. Turn them as they heat up. It should only take a few seconds to get the tortillas warm enough to bend without cracking. Lay each warm tortilla on a clean surface and fill each one with equal portions of grilled steak. Position the steak near the bottom edge of the burrito with about a 1-inch "margin."

6. Take half of the sautéed peppers and onions and split it between the two burritos, laying it on the steak.

7. Roll the burrito by folding the bottom up and over the filling. Fold in the sides, and then roll the filling up over twice, being careful to make a neat little package.

8. Rub 1 teaspoon of vegetable oil over the entire surface of each burrito.

9. Put the burritos, seam side down, back on your barbecue grill set on medium heat for 1 to 2 minutes. When the bottom of the burrito begins to char, turn the burritos over. By now the tortilla should be stiff and crunchy making it easy to roll the burrito over without the filling falling out. Grill the tops of the burritos for 1 to 2 minutes more, or until the surface begins to char.

10. Transfer the burritos from the grill to two serving plates with the seam side down. Coat the top of each burrito with 1 to 1½ tablespoons of barbecue sauce.

11. Split the remaining peppers and onions and spread them over the top of the two burritos.

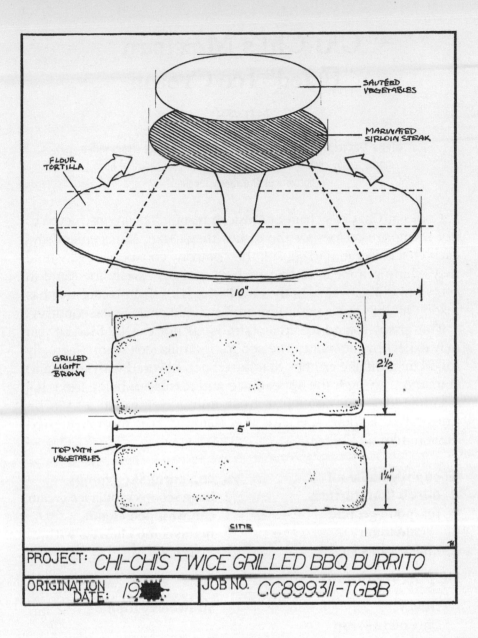

SAUTÉED VEGETABLES

MARINATED SIRLOIN STEAK

FLOUR TORTILLA

10"

GRILLED LIGHT BROWN

2½"

5"

TOP WITH VEGETABLES

1¼"

SIDE

PROJECT: CHI-CHI'S TWICE GRILLED BBQ BURRITO

ORIGINATION DATE: 19██

JOB NO. CC899311-TGBB

97

✳ Chi-Chi's Mexican "Fried" Ice Cream

Serves 2

Menu Description: "Our specialty! French Vanilla ice cream with a crunchy, crispy cinnamon coating. Served with your choice of honey, chocolate or strawberry topping."

Cooks at Chi-Chi's chain of Mexican restaurants are instructed to *not* memorize recipes for the dishes they make. Management says each chef is required to consult the company cookbooks every time they whip up a meal, so that each dish tastes exactly the same in every Chi-Chi's any time of the day. Perhaps it's that practice that has made Chi-Chi's the largest Mexican restaurant chain in the country.

This crispy-coated ice cream sundae is not exactly fried as you may expect by the name. The scoop of vanilla ice cream is actually rolled in cornflake crumbs that have been flavored with sugar and cinnamon, giving it the appearance and texture of being fried. It's a simple idea that tastes just great, and is well worth a try. Chi-Chi's calls this their "specialty" and claims it's the most requested dessert item on the menu.

½ cup vegetable oil	¼ cup cornflake crumbs
2 6-inch flour tortillas	2 large scoops vanilla ice cream
½ teaspoon ground cinnamon	1 can whipped cream
2 tablespoons sugar	2 maraschino cherries with stems

Topping (optional)

Honey	Strawberry topping
Chocolate syrup	

1. Prepare each tortilla by frying it in the hot oil in a frying pan over medium/high heat. Fry each side of the tortilla for about 1 minute until crispy. Drain the tortillas on paper towels.
2. Combine the cinnamon and sugar in a small bowl.

3. Sprinkle half of the cinnamon mixture over both sides of the fried tortillas, coating evenly. Not all of the sugar mixture will stick to the tortillas, and that's okay.
4. Combine the other half of the cinnamon mixture with the corn-flake crumbs in another small bowl. Pour the cornflake mixture into a wide, shallow bowl or onto a plate.

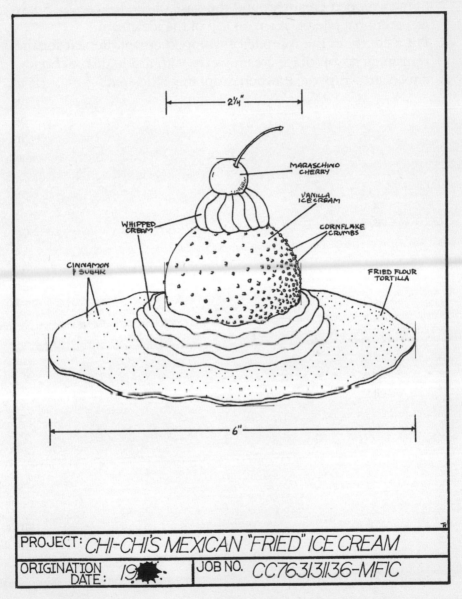

PROJECT: *CHI-CHI'S MEXICAN "FRIED" ICE CREAM*

ORIGINATION DATE: *19___.* JOB NO. *CC7631311.36-MFIC*

5. Place a large scoop of ice cream in the cornflake crumbs, and with your hands roll the ice cream around until the entire surface is evenly coated with cornflake crumbs. You should not be able to see the ice cream.
6. Place the ice cream scoop on the center of a cinnamon/sugar-coated tortilla.
7. Spray whipped cream around the base of the ice cream. Spray an additional pile of cream on top of the ice cream.
8. Put a cherry in the top pile of whipped cream. Repeat for the remaining scoop of ice cream. Serve with a side dish of honey, chocolate syrup, or strawberry topping, if desired.

✳ Chili's Grilled Caribbean Salad

Serves 2 as an entree

Menu Description: "Grilled, marinated chicken breast, mixed greens, pico de gallo, pineapple chunks, tortilla strips & honey-lime dressing."

Larry Levine started building his chain of Chili's restaurants in Dallas in 1975. At that time Chili's was basically a hamburger joint with a gourmet touch, dining room service and booze. Even though the menu then offered only eleven items, the restaurant was so popular that throngs of hungry customers waited patiently in lines extending into the parking lots. This caught the eye of the persuasive restaurateur Norman Brinker, who, in 1983, convinced Larry to sell his chain of Chili's restaurants, which by then had grown to a total of thirty.

Before Norman had stepped into the picture, more than 80 percent of Chili's business was in hamburgers. Today a much larger menu reflects the current trends in food, and salads are some of the best-selling items. These days the Grilled Caribbean Salad with the tasty honey-lime dressing is the salad of choice.

Honey-Lime Dressing

¼ cup Grey Poupon Dijon mustard
¼ cup honey
1½ tablespoons sugar
1 tablespoon sesame oil
1½ tablespoons apple cider vinegar
1½ teaspoons lime juice

Blend all the ingredients in a small bowl with an electric mixer. Cover and chill.

101

Pico de Gallo

2 medium tomatoes, diced
½ cup diced Spanish onion
2 teaspoons chopped fresh
    jalapeño pepper, seeded
    and de-ribbed

2 teaspoons finely minced
    fresh cilantro*
Pinch of salt

Combine all the ingredients in a small bowl. Cover and chill.

Salad

4 boneless, skinless chicken
    breast halves
½ cup teriyaki marinade,
    store bought or your own
    (page 305)
4 cups chopped iceberg
    lettuce

4 cups chopped green leaf
    lettuce
1 cup chopped red cabbage
1 5.5-ounce can pineapple
    chunks in juice, drained
10 tortilla chips

1. Marinate the chicken in the teriyaki for at least 2 hours. You can use a resealable plastic bag for this. Put the chicken into the bag and pour in the marinade, then toss it into the fridge.
2. Prepare the barbecue or preheat a stovetop grill. Grill the chicken for 4 to 5 minutes per side or until done.
3. Toss the lettuce and cabbage together, then divide the greens into two large individual-serving salad bowls.
4. Divide the pico de gallo and pour it in two even portions over the greens.
5. Divide the pineapple and sprinkle it on the salads.
6. Break the tortilla chips into large chunks and sprinkle half on each salad.
7. Slice the grilled chicken breasts into thin strips, and spread half the strips onto each salad.
8. Pour the dressing into two small bowls and serve with the salads.

*Found in the produce section; also known as fresh coriander and Chinese parsley.

✳ Chili's Fajitas for Two

Serves 2 as an entree

Menu Description: "A pound of steak, chicken or combination on a sizzling skillet. Peppers available w/Fajitas upon request."

Chili's is perhaps the restaurant most responsible for introducing the famous finger food known as fajitas to the mass market. Company CEO Norman Brinker discovered the dish at a small restaurant on a visit to San Antonio, Texas. When Chili's put the item on its menu in the early eighties, sales immediately jumped a whopping 25 percent. One company spokesperson told *Spirit* magazine, "I remember walking into one of the restaurants after we added them to the menu and all I could see were wisps of steam coming up from the tables. That revolutionized Chili's."

Today Chili's serves more than 2 million pounds of fajitas a year. If all of the flour tortillas served with those fajitas were laid end-to-end, they'd stretch from New York to New Zealand, on the other side of the earth!

Today just about every American knows what fajitas are—the Southwestern-style grilled chicken, beef, or seafood, served sizzling on a cast iron skillet. And everyone has their own method of arranging the meat and onions and peppers in a soft tortilla with globs of pico de gallo, cheese, guacamole, lettuce, sour cream, and salsa. The tough part is trying to roll the thing up and take a bite ever so gracefully without squeezing half of the filling out the backside of the tortilla onto the plate, splattering your clean clothes, while goo goes dripping down your chin. This recipe is guaranteed to be as delicious and messy as the original.

Marinade

¼ cup fresh lime juice
⅓ cup water
2 tablespoons vegetable oil
1 large clove garlic, pressed
3 teaspoons vinegar
2 teaspoons soy sauce
½ teaspoon liquid smoke

1 teaspoon salt
½ teaspoon chili powder
½ teaspoon cayenne
   pepper
¼ teaspoon ground black
   pepper
Dash onion powder

2 boneless, skinless chicken
   breast halves *or* 1 pound
   top sirloin *or* a combination of 1 chicken breast
   half and ½ pound sirloin
1 Spanish onion, sliced

1 tablespoon vegetable oil
1 teaspoon soy sauce
2 tablespoons water
½ teaspoon lime juice
Dash ground black pepper
Dash salt

On the Side

½ cup pico de gallo (page 102)
½ cup grated Cheddar cheese
½ cup guacamole
½ cup sour cream

1 cup shredded lettuce
6 to 8 6-inch flour tortillas
Salsa

1. Combine all of the ingredients for the marinade in a small bowl. Soak your choice of meat in the marinade for at least 2 hours. If you are just using the sirloin, let it marinate overnight, if possible.
2. When the meat has marinated, preheat your barbecue or stove-top grill to high.
3. Preheat a skillet over medium/high heat. Sauté the onion slices in the oil for 5 minutes. Combine the soy sauce, water, and lime juice in a small bowl and pour it over the onions. Add the black pepper and continue to sauté until the onions are translucent and dark on the edges (4 to 5 more minutes). Salt to taste.
4. While the onions are sautéing, grill the meat for 4 to 5 minutes per side or until done.
5. While the meat and onions are cooking, heat up another skillet (cast iron if you have one) over high heat. This will be your sizzling serving pan.

6. When the meat is done remove it from the grill and slice it into thin strips.
7. Remove the extra pan from the heat and dump the onions and any liquid into it. If you've made it hot enough the onions should sizzle. Add the meat to the pan and serve immediately with pico de gallo, Cheddar cheese, guacamole, and sour cream arranged on a separate plate on a bed of shredded lettuce. Steam the tortillas in a moist towel in the microwave for 30 seconds and serve on the side. Serve salsa also, if desired.

Assemble fajitas by putting the meat into a tortilla along with your choice of condiments. Roll up the tortilla and scarf out.

Tidbits

At Chili's, bell peppers are optional with this dish. If you like peppers, combine a small slice of green or red bell pepper with the onion, and saute the vegetables together. Follow the rest of the steps as described.

✳ Chili's Peanut Buttercup Cheesecake

Serves 10

Menu Description: "Chocolate & vanilla marbled cheesecake on a chocolate cookie crust, topped w/fudge & Reese's Peanut Butter Cup pieces."

If I had to pick one person in the restaurant business with the most respected and distinguished career, it would have to be Norman Brinker. The 65-year-old CEO of Brinker International is still building on a success story that spans four decades, and recently detailed his life in an autobiography, *On the Brink*. Back in the fifties, Norman took a job with Robert Peterson, who had just a few years earlier opened the first Jack-in-the-Box in San Diego, California. By the age of 34, Norman owned 20 percent of Jack-in-the-Box, giving him enough capital to set out on his own venture. In 1964 he opened a fifties-style coffee shop in downtown Dallas called Brinks. He sold that eatery a year later for $6,000 and sank that cash into a new chain that would become one of his most successful ventures. Norman opened the first Steak and Ale in 1966, took the chain public in 1971, then 10 years later sold the whole kit-and-caboodle for $100 million to the Pillsbury Company (that's some serious dough, boy). Pillsbury kept him on to run the operation, but Norman needed new action. In 1983, he purchased Chili's from founder Larry Levine and within 12 years built the chain into a billion-dollar company. Today Norman continues to watch Brinker International grow as new concepts like Cozymel's and Romano's Macaroni Grill are added to his long list of restaurant chain successes.

Speaking of rich, here's a tasty dessert for anyone who digs cheesecake and peanut butter cups. Use an 8-inch springform pan for this recipe if you have one. If not, you can also use two 9-inch pie pans and make two smaller cheesecakes. For the Oreo cookie crumbs, you can crumble three Oreo cookies, after removing the filling, or you can find packaged Oreo crumbs in the baking section of your supermarket near the graham cracker crumbs.

1 cup graham cracker crumbs	3 eggs
¼ cup Oreo chocolate cookie crumbs (3 cookies with filling removed)	1 cup sour cream
	1 cup sugar
	1½ teaspoons vanilla
⅓ cup butter, melted	¼ cup chocolate syrup
¼ cup smooth peanut butter (not chunky)	1 cup fudge topping
	4 chilled regular-size Reese's peanut butter cups (not bite-size)
3 8-ounce packages cream cheese, softened	

1. Preheat the oven to 375 degrees F.
2. In a medium bowl combine the graham cracker crumbs, chocolate cookie crumbs, and melted butter.
3. Press the crumbs firmly over just the bottom of an 8-inch springform pan. Bake for 6 to 8 minutes.
4. When the crust is cool, spread the peanut butter in a circle in the center of the crust. (You may soften the peanut butter for 30 seconds in the microwave to make it easier to spread.) You don't need to spread the peanut butter to the edge—leave about an inch margin all around.
5. You'll need two separate bowls for the two fillings, one larger than the other. In the larger bowl, with an electric mixer, beat together the cream cheese, eggs, sour cream, sugar, and vanilla until smooth.
6. Remove 1 cup of the cream cheese mixture and pour it into the smaller bowl. Add the chocolate syrup to this mixture and combine.
7. Pour the large bowl of filling into the pan and spread it evenly over the crust.
8. Pour the chocolate filling onto the other filling and spread it out. Using the tip of a knife, swirl the chocolate into the white filling beneath it. A couple of passes should be enough.
9. Lower the oven temperature to 350 degrees F. Bake the cheesecake for 70 to 80 minutes or until it becomes firm in the center. Remove from the oven and allow it to cool.
10. When the cheesecake is completely cool, soften the fudge topping in a double boiler or the microwave for about 45 seconds, then spread it out evenly over the cheesecake. Be sure to cover the entire surface of the filling.

11. Unwrap the peanut butter cups and chop them into small chunks.
12. Sprinkle the peanut butter cup pieces and any crumbs over the top of the cheesecake. Chill.
13. Slice the cake 5 times through the middle to make 10 slices.

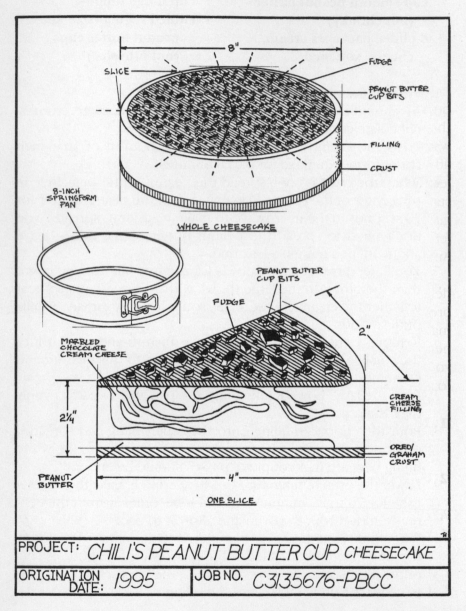

8"

SLICE

FUDGE

PEANUT BUTTER
CUP BITS

FILLING

CRUST

8-INCH
SPRINGFORM
PAN

WHOLE CHEESECAKE

PEANUT BUTTER
CUP BITS

FUDGE

2"

MARBLED
CHOCOLATE
CREAM CHEESE

CREAM
CHEESE
FILLING

2¼"

OREO/
GRAHAM
CRUST

PEANUT
BUTTER

4"

ONE SLICE

PROJECT: CHILI'S PEANUT BUTTER CUP CHEESECAKE

ORIGINATION DATE: 1995

JOB NO. C3135676-PBCC

✳ Cracker Barrel Hash Brown Casserole

Serves 4 to 6 as a side dish

Menu Description: "Made from scratch in our kitchens using fresh Grade A Fancy Russet potatoes, fresh chopped onion, natural Colby cheese and spices. Baked fresh all day long."

In the late sixties Dan Evins was a Shell Oil "jobber" looking for a new way to market gasoline. He wanted to create a special place that would arouse curiosity, and would pull travelers off the highways. In 1969 he opened the first Cracker Barrel just off Interstate 40 in Lebanon, Tennessee, offering gas, country-style food, and a selection of antiques for sale. Today there are over 260 stores in 22 states, with each restaurant still designed as a country reststop and gift store. In fact, those stores (which carry an average of 4,500 different items apiece) have made Cracker Barrel the largest retailer of American-made finished crafts in the United States.

Those who know Cracker Barrel well love the restaurant for its delicious home-style breakfasts. This casserole, made with hash browns, Colby cheese, milk, beef stock, and spices is served with many of the classic breakfast dishes at the restaurant. The recipe here is designed for a skillet that is also safe to put in the oven. If you don't have one of those, you can easily transfer the casserole to a baking dish after it is done cooking on the stove.

1 26-ounce bag frozen country-style hash browns	½ cup beef stock or canned broth
2 cups shredded Colby cheese	2 tablespoons butter, melted
¼ cup minced onion	Dash garlic powder
1 cup milk	1 teaspoon salt
	¼ teaspoon ground black pepper

1. Preheat the oven to 425 degrees F.
2. Combine the frozen hash browns, cheese, and onion in a large bowl.

3. Combine the milk, beef stock, half the melted butter, the garlic powder, salt, and black pepper in another bowl. Mix until well blended, then pour the mixture over the hash browns and mix well.
4. Heat the remaining butter in a large, ovenproof skillet over high heat.
5. When the skillet is hot, spoon in the hash brown mixture. Cook the hash browns, stirring occasionally, until hot and all of the cheese has melted (about 7 minutes).
6. Put the skillet into the oven and bake for 45 to 60 minutes or until the surface of the hash browns is dark brown.

Tidbits

If your skillet isn't ovenproof (because it has a plastic handle, for example), you can also spoon the potatoes into a glass 9 × 9-inch baking dish and microwave the potatoes until they are hot and the cheese has melted. Then put that baking dish into the 425 degrees F oven until the surface of the hash browns has browned.

If you can't find Colby cheese, you can also use Cheddar cheese for this recipe. Colby, however, is preferred.

✳ Cracker Barrel
Eggs-in-the-Basket

Serves 1 (can be doubled)

Menu Description: "Two slices of sourdough bread grilled with an egg in the middle, served with thick sliced bacon or smoked sausage patties and fried apples or hash brown casserole."

Breakfast is a popular meal at Cracker Barrel restaurants. Just to prove it, the restaurant has some amazing statistics printed on the back of their breakfast menus:

"Each Spring 607,142 Sugar Maple Trees must be tapped to produce enough pure maple syrup for our guests.

"It takes 5,615,00,000 (THAT'S BILLION!) coffee beans each year to satisfy our guests' needs for coffee. Each tree produces only 1 pound of coffee per year . . . that's 1,560,000 trees."

And if you've ever wondered who the man is on the restaurant's logo:

"Uncle Herschel, the country gentleman on our logo, really is the uncle of Cracker Barrel president, Dan Evins."

This recipe is from an old-fashioned egg-in-the-hole meal that I used to make all the time as a kid. Heck, I thought my family had invented it! I was surprised to see this offered on the Cracker Barrel menu, and then I was thrilled to find it tasted just like the homemade version we used to make years ago. This version of the Cracker Barrel classic goes great with the Hash Brown Casserole recipe (page 109). If you're making this for more than just one person, the recipe is easily doubled or quadrupled.

2 thick slices sourdough bread	2 eggs
2 tablespoons butter, softened	Salt to taste

On the Side

Sausage	Thick-sliced bacon

1. Heat a large frying pan or griddle over medium heat.
2. Spread the butter evenly over one face of each slice of bread.
3. Use a biscuit cutter or any jar or container you can find with a diameter of about 2¼ inches to cut a circle out of the center of each slice of bread.

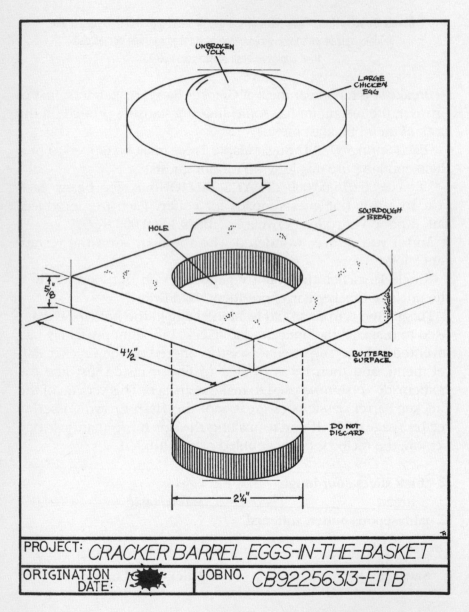

4. Grill the bread and the hole you cut out, butter side down, in the hot pan for 2 minutes or until it just starts to turn brown.
5. Drop a little butter in the hole of each slice of bread, then carefully crack an egg into each hole. Be sure not to break the yolks. Salt lightly.
6. When the eggs have cooked for 1 to 2 minutes, carefully flip each one over without breaking the yolks or flinging raw egg goo all over the stovetop. Also, flip the cut-out "holes."
7. Cook for another minute or so until the eggs are cooked the way you like them. Serve the eggs, grilled bread, and "holes" with hash browns or Hash Brown Casserole, and bacon or sausage.

✳ Cracker Barrel
Chicken & Dumplins

Serves 4 as an entree

Menu Description: *"We use only the 'best of the breast' chicken tenderloin in our recipe. Our dumplins are made from scratch, then hand rolled and cut into strips before simmering to perfection in chicken stock."*

By 1977 there were 13 Cracker Barrel stores located in Georgia and Tennessee, with all of them based on founder Dan Evins' original concept of a restaurant and store built around gasoline pumps. But with the oil embargo and energy crisis of the mid-seventies, Cracker Barrel started building stores that did not offer gas. Soon all of the original 13 stores were converted so that today not one Cracker Barrel lets you "filler-up" while you fill yourself up.

Another old-time favorite at Cracker Barrel is the Chicken & Dumplins on the lunch and dinner menu. The nice thing about this version of the popular classic dish is that it creates its own tasty gravy. As the "dumplins" dissolve some, the flour thickens the stock into a creamy sauce. Just remember to let your dough rest a bit before rolling it to cut out the dumplins. This will allow the gluten in the flour to work much better. Use extra flour on your cutting board and rolling pin if the dough is too tacky, and try not to roll the dough too thin.

Chicken and broth

3 quarts water	1 bay leaf
1 3- to 4-pound chicken, cut up	4 to 6 whole parsley leaves
1½ teaspoons salt	1 teaspoon coarsely ground black pepper
1 small onion, sliced	1 tablespoon lemon juice
2 stalks celery, chopped	
1 clove garlic, peeled and quartered	

"Dumplins"

2 cups all-purpose flour	1¼ teaspoons salt
1 tablespoon baking powder	1 cup plus 2 tablespoons milk

1. Bring the water to a boil in a large pot. Add the chicken, 1 teaspoon of salt, onion, celery, garlic, bay leaf, and parsley to the pot. Reduce the heat to simmer and cook the chicken, uncovered, for 2 hours. The liquid will reduce by about one third.
2. When the chicken has cooked, remove it from the pot and set it aside. Strain the stock to remove all the vegetables and floating scum. You only want the stock and the chicken, so toss everything else out.
3. Pour 1½ quarts (6 cups) of the stock back into the pot (keep the leftover stock, if any, for another recipe—it can be frozen). You may also want to use a smaller pot or a large saucepan for this. Add coarsely ground pepper, the remaining ½ teaspoon salt, and the lemon juice, then reheat the stock over medium heat while preparing the dumplins.
4. For dumplins, combine the flour, baking powder, 1¼ teaspoons salt, and milk in a medium bowl. Stir well until smooth, then let the dough rest for to 5 to 10 minutes. Roll the dough out onto a floured surface to about a ½-inch thickness.
5. Cut the dough into ½-inch squares and drop each square into the simmering stock. Use all of the dough. The dumplins will first swell and then slowly shrink as they partially dissolve to thicken the stock into a white gravy. Simmer for 20 to 30 minutes until thick. Stir often.
6. While the stock is thickening, the chicken will have become cool enough to handle. Tear all the meat from the bones and remove the skin. Cut the chicken meat into bite-size or a little bigger than bite-size pieces and drop them into the pot. Discard the skin and bones. Continue to simmer the chicken and dumplins for another 5 to 10 minutes, but don't stir too vigorously or the chicken will shred and fall apart. You want big chunks of chicken in the end.
7. When the gravy has reached the desired consistency, ladle four portions onto plates and serve hot. Serve with your choice of steamed vegetables, if desired.

✳ Denny's Scram Slam

Serves 2

Menu Description: "Three eggs scrambled with Cheddar cheese,
mushrooms, green peppers and onions, then topped with diced tomatoes.
Served with hashed browns, sausage, bacon and choice of toast,
Homestyle buttermilk biscuit or English muffin."

In 1953, Harold Butler realized his dream of opening a donut shop. The little shop in Lakewood, California was called Danny's Donuts, and Harold's philosophy was simple: "We're going to serve the best cup of coffee; make the best donuts; give the best service; keep everything spotless; offer the best value; and stay open 24 hours a day."

That little donut store made $120,000 in its first year—a good bit of change for any restaurant in 1953. When customers requested more than fried dough with a hole in the middle, Harold began offering sandwiches, breakfasts, and other meals, and in 1954 changed the name to Danny's Coffee Shops. The name of the chain would eventually change again, this time to Denny's—now the nation's largest full-service restaurant chain.

In 1977, Denny's introduced the Grand Slam Breakfast—a value-priced breakfast that included eggs, sausage, bacon, and pancakes. Later, the successful Grand Slam Breakfast specials expanded to included other variations including the French Slam, Southern Slam, and the Scram Slam, the last a popular vegetable-and-scrambled-egg creation you can now make for yourself.

1 slice white onion, diced (¼ cup)	1½ tablespoons butter
¼ green bell pepper, diced (¼ cup)	6 eggs, beaten
4 mushrooms, sliced (1 cup)	1 cup shredded Cheddar cheese
	Salt
	½ tomato, chopped

116

On the Side

Bacon   **Hash browns**
Sausage

1. In a small skillet, sauté the onion, green pepper, and mushrooms in 1 tablespoon of the butter over medium heat for about 5 minutes or until the mushrooms are tender.
2. In another larger skillet over medium heat, melt the remaining ½ tablespoon butter. Add the beaten eggs. Stir the eggs as they cook to scramble them.
3. When the eggs have cooked for 5 to 7 minutes and are no longer runny, add the cheese and stir. Add the sautéed onions, green pepper, and mushrooms along with a dash of salt and cook the eggs until done.
4. Divide the eggs onto two plates and sprinkle chopped tomatoes over each helping. Serve with bacon, sausage, and hash browns on the side.

✳ Denny's Moons Over
My Hammy

Serves 1 (can be doubled)

Menu Description: "The supreme ham and egg sandwich,
made with Swiss and American cheese on grilled sourdough.
Served with choice of hashed browns or French fries."

With its goofy-yet-memorable name, Moons Over My Hammy is
a delicious and versatile scrambled egg sandwich that can be eaten
for breakfast with hash browns on the side, or for lunch with a side
of French fries. When you get the sourdough bread for this recipe,
try to find a good-quality loaf with large slices.

Butter, softened
2 eggs, beaten
Salt
2 ounces deli-sliced ham
2 slices sourdough bread

1 to 2 slices processed Swiss
   cheese (Kraft Singles)
1 to 2 slices American cheese
   (Kraft Singles)

On the side

Hash browns   French fries

1. Put two medium-size skillets over medium heat. In one skillet,
   add a little butter and scramble the two eggs. Salt the eggs to
   taste. In the other skillet, brown the stack of sliced ham without separating the slices.
2. When the stack of ham slices has browned a bit on both sides, remove it from the pan. Butter one side of each slice of sourdough
   bread and put one slice into the pan, buttered side down, to grill.
3. Immediately put the slice(s) of Swiss cheese onto the face-up,
   unbuttered side of the bread that is grilling.
4. Stack the heated ham slices on the Swiss cheese.
5. Scoop the scrambled eggs out of the other pan with a large
   spatula and place them on the ham.
6. Place the slice(s) of American cheese on the eggs.
7. Top off the sandwich with the remaining slice of sourdough
   bread. Make sure the unbuttered side faces the cheese.

8. By this time the bread touching the pan should be grilled to a golden brown. Carefully flip the sandwich over and grill the other side for about 2 minutes or until brown.
9. Slice the sandwich diagonally through the middle and serve with hash browns or French fries on the side.

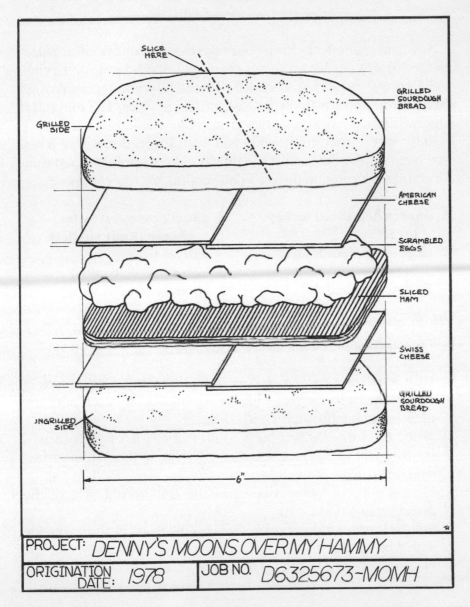

SLICE HERE

GRILLED SOURDOUGH BREAD

GRILLED SIDE

AMERICAN CHEESE

SCRAMBLED EGGS

SLICED HAM

SWISS CHEESE

GRILLED SOURDOUGH BREAD

UNGRILLED SIDE

6"

PROJECT: DENNY'S MOONS OVER MY HAMMY

ORIGINATION DATE: 1978   JOB NO. D6325673-MOMH

✳ Denny's The Super Bird

Serves 1 (can be doubled)

Menu Description: "A Denny's original. Sliced turkey breast
with Swiss cheese, bacon and tomato on grilled sourdough.
Served with French fries and pickle chips."

Now you can munch down your own clone of this popular palate
pleaser, The Super Bird, a cross between a grilled cheese and a club,
and Denny's top-selling sandwich. When shopping for sourdough
bread, try to find a high-quality loaf with large slices. The thin-sliced
turkey breast is best purchased at your market's deli service
counter where they cut it while you wait. If you don't have a service counter like this near you, you can use the prepackaged thin-
sliced meats located in the cold deli section. Or you can move.

3 ounces deli-sliced turkey
  breast
2 large slices sourdough
  bread
  Butter, softened

2 slices processed Swiss
  cheese (Kraft Singles)
  Salt
2 slices bacon, cooked
2 slices tomato

On the Side

French fries

Pickles

1. Heat a skillet or frying pan over medium heat. Grill the stack of
   turkey breast in the pan without separating the stack until the
   meat is golden brown on both sides.
2. While the turkey is browning, butter one side of each slice of
   sourdough bread. Place one slice of bread in the pan, buttered
   side down.
3. Place a slice of Swiss cheese on the unbuttered side of the
   bread grilling in the pan.
4. Put the stack of turkey breast slices on the Swiss cheese. Sprinkle
   with a bit of salt.
5. Place the cooked bacon on the turkey breast.

6. Stack the tomato slices on the bacon next.
7. Top off the sandwich with the remaining slice of sourdough bread. Be sure to place the bread with the unbuttered side facing the tomato slices.

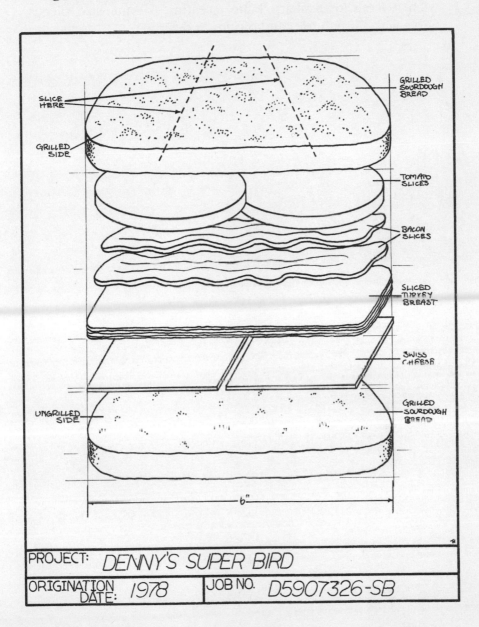

SLICE HERE

GRILLED SIDE

GRILLED SOURDOUGH BREAD

TOMATO SLICES

BACON SLICES

SLICED TURKEY BREAST

SWISS CHEESE

UNGRILLED SIDE

GRILLED SOURDOUGH BREAD

6"

PROJECT: DENNY'S SUPER BIRD

ORIGINATION DATE: 1978

JOB NO. D5907326-SB

8. When the slice of bread on the bottom has grilled until golden brown, carefully flip the sandwich over to grill the other slice.

9. After about 2 minutes, when the bread has grilled to a golden brown, remove the sandwich from the pan and slice the sandwich twice with a sharp knife, creating 3 equal-size pieces. Serve with French fries and pickles, if desired.

✳ Dive!
Carrot Chips

Serves 4 as an appetizer or snack

Menu Description: "Crisp, lightly fried carrots, choice of two dips."

In 1992, Steven Spielberg organized a search for a hoagie like those he remembered from his childhood in Phoenix, Arizona. The famed director sent his assistants out to search L.A. for the perfect submarine sandwich, and from the 20 sandwiches brought back to him, not one passed the test. Former chairman of Walt Disney Studios and close friend Jeffrey Katzenberg was in on the taste test that day and agreed that most of the sandwiches were either too soggy or too leathery. The two began tossing the idea around of opening their own restaurant to reinvent the submarine sandwich with fresh baked bread and unique combinations of ingredients—like what Spago's and California Pizza Kitchen were doing with pizza. Partnered with Mark and Larry Levy of Levy Restaurants, the two movie moguls tasted over 100 sandwich recipes before finding two dozen they liked. A year of planning went by to build a deep-sea theme around the recipes, and in 1994, the first Dive! restaurant opened in L.A.

In addition to the gourmet sandwiches on the menu, Dive! features pastas, salads, burgers, and delicious appetizers like carrot chips complete with your choice of dipping sauces. Because the carrots need to be sliced no thicker than $\frac{1}{16}$ inch, you'll probably have to use a thin-slicing machine such as a mandoline for this recipe. I tried doing it by hand, and it's practically impossible to get the carrots a uniform thickness without using a gadget.

6 carrots	**4 to 6 cups canola oil**

On the Side

Barbecue sauce (commercial brand, or see pages 300–303)	Cajun Mayonnaise Dipping Sauce (follows)
	White Cheddar Dipping Sauce (follows)

1. Peel the carrots, then slice them crosswise in half. Use a slicer to make lengthwise, thin slices of carrot, no more than $\frac{1}{16}$ inch thick.
2. Heat the oil in a deep pot or deep fryer to 350 degrees F.
3. Drop a handful of carrot slices at a time into the hot oil. Fry the carrots for 10 to 15 seconds or until they turn a dark brown. Remove the carrots from the oil; drain and cool the carrots on paper towels, then put them in a large, shallow bowl. Serve with ketchup, a store-bought dip (such as barbecue sauce), or your choice of dipping sauces from the recipes here.

Cajun Mayonnaise Dipping Sauce

½ cup mayonnaise
1 teaspoon lemon juice
¼ teaspoon cayenne
   pepper
⅛ teaspoon garlic powder
⅛ teaspoon onion powder
⅛ teaspoon ground black
   pepper
⅛ teaspoon paprika
⅛ teaspoon dried thyme
Dash salt
Pinch dried oregano

1. Combine all of the ingredients in a small bowl.
2. Cover and refrigerate for several hours or overnight before serving.

White Cheddar Dipping Sauce

½ cup heavy cream
1 to 2 ounces white Cheddar
   cheese, grated or
   chopped
1 tablespoon butter

1. Combine all of the ingredients in a small saucepan over medium heat.
2. Bring the mixture to a boil, then reduce the heat and simmer for 10 minutes. By then the sauce should have thickened. Serve hot.

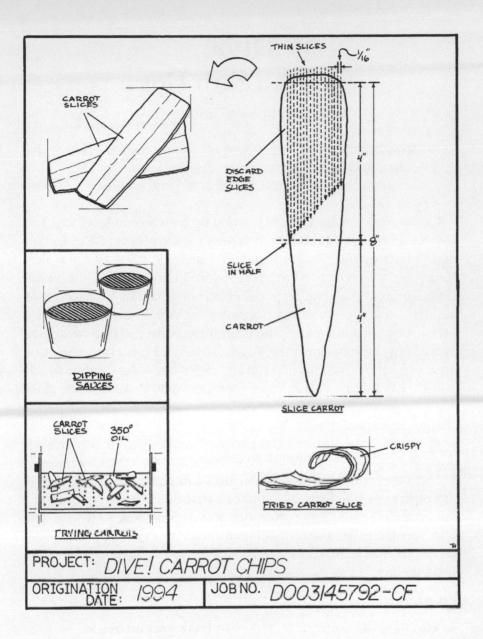

CARROT SLICES

THIN SLICES

1/16"

DISCARD EDGE SLICES

4"

8"

SLICE IN HALF

4"

CARROT

SLICE CARROT

DIPPING SAUCES

CARROT SLICES

350° OIL

FRYING CARROTS

CRISPY

FRIED CARROT SLICE

PROJECT: *DIVE! CARROT CHIPS*

ORIGINATION DATE: *1994*

JOB NO. *D003145792-CF*

125

✳ Dive!
Sicilian Sub Rosa

Serves 1 (can be doubled)

Menu Description: "Our traditional sub with capocollo, mortadella, Genoa salami, prosciutto ham, provolone cheese, roasted red peppers, fresh basil, lettuce, sliced tomato, onions and vinaigrette. Served hot or cold."

Casino magnate Steve Wynn teamed up with Steven Spielberg, Jeffrey Katzenberg, and the Levy Brothers for the second Dive! restaurant, which opened in Las Vegas in March of 1995. Like the first restaurant, which opened the year before in Los Angeles, the Vegas Dive! features Spielbergian special effects designed by Hollywood set builders, such as bubbling portholes, spinning gauges, working periscopes, steaming pipes, and a simulated dive run by a computer every hour. Driving down the Vegas "strip" you can't miss the giant nose of a submarine crashing through a 30-foot wall of water, which pumps 100 gallons of water per foot per minute down thick glass window panes. A pool below explodes with synchronized depth charges that splash passersby at random intervals. Back inside, if you look carefully, you can see the partners' initials stenciled on torpedoes hanging high over the heads of diners.

The Dive! concept was built around submarine sandwiches and the Sicilian Sub Rosa is its signature traditional Italian submarine sandwich. It's said to be cofounder Steven Spielberg's favorite and now you can make a version all your own. Try to get all of the meat sliced fresh at a full-service deli counter, if you have one at your supermarket.

Vinaigrette

¼ cup light olive oil
1 tablespoon red wine
vinegar
½ teaspoon lemon juice

Dash ground black
pepper
Dash salt
Dash garlic powder

126

1 handful of thinly sliced and separated red onion rings (about ⅛ onion)
1 7-inch baguette
1 leaf green leaf lettuce
1 ounce deli-sliced prosciutto
1 ounce deli-sliced capocollo
1 ounce deli-sliced mortadella
1 ounce deli-sliced Genoa salami
1 ounce deli-sliced provolone cheese
1 ounce roasted red peppers (canned or homemade, see "Tidbits")
4 to 5 small fresh basil leaves
3 tomato slices

1. Mix the vinaigrette ingredients together in a small bowl and add the sliced and separated red onion rings to the bowl. Let the onions marinate for at least a couple hours. Overnight is even better.
2. When the onions are ready, slice open the baguette, without cutting all of the way through. Brush a generous amount of the vinaigrette on the faces of the baguette.
3. Spread the leaf of lettuce on the baguette.
4. Arrange the prosciutto over the lettuce.
5. Next, stack the capocollo.
6. On the capocollo goes the mortadella.
7. Then the Genoa salami.
8. Next is the provolone.
9. Arrange the roasted red peppers on the provolone cheese.
10. Spread the fresh basil leaves on the sandwich next.
11. Arrange the sliced tomatoes on the basil leaves.
12. Remove the red onions from the vinaigrette and spread them on top of the tomatoes.
13. Close the sandwich and use toothpicks to keep it that way to serve. If you want the sandwich hot, before you close it, put it in a preheated 450 degree F oven for 4 minutes and then broil it for 2 minutes. The cheese should melt slightly and the bread will become slightly browned. Slice the sandwich in half before serving.

Tidbits

Canned roasted peppers are usually pretty good, but if you want to make great roasted peppers yourself, put a whole red bell pepper directly on the burner of a gas stove set to medium heat or on a pan in an oven set to broil. Turn the pepper often with tongs until most of the skin of the pepper is charred black. Immediately drop the pepper into a bowl of ice water and carefully peel the skin away. Remove the seeds, chop the remaining pepper into slices for your sandwich and store the leftovers in a sealed container in the refrigerator.

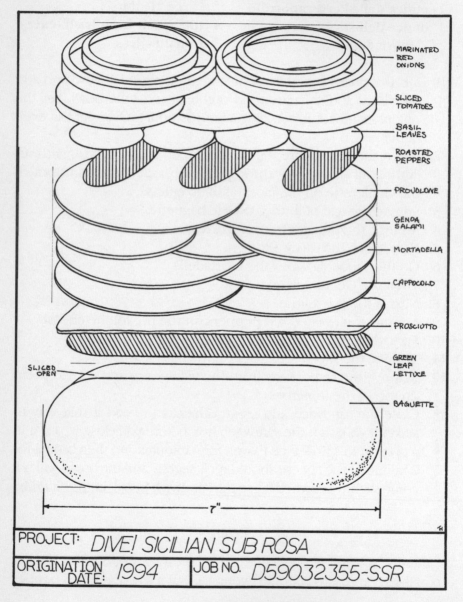

MARINATED RED ONIONS

SLICED TOMATOES

BASIL LEAVES

ROASTED PEPPERS

PROVOLONE

GENOA SALAMI

MORTADELLA

CAPPOCOLO

PROSCIUTTO

GREEN LEAF LETTUCE

BAGUETTE

SLICED OPEN

7"

PROJECT: DIVE! SICILIAN SUB ROSA

ORIGINATION DATE: 1994   JOB NO. D59032355-SSR

✳ Dive! Brick Oven Mushroom and Turkey Cheese Sub

Serves 1 (can be doubled)

Menu Description: "Our fresh roasted turkey, brick oven roasted seasonal mushrooms with white cheddar cheese and melted Swiss cheese. Served hot."

Although not intended to be a restaurant where sightseers are encouraged to catch a glimpse of celebrities, many stars have been spotted at the L.A. location of this trendy new theme eatery. Through the "hatch" have walked the likes of Candice Bergen, Warren Beatty, Michael Keaton, Tom Hanks, Michael Douglas, and Rob Reiner. Pierce Brosnan and Henry Winkler have become regulars, and for some time cofounder Steven Spielberg could be seen eating there weekly. At least ten new Dive! locations are being planned for additional U.S. and international markets including New York, Chicago, Mexico, and Japan.

For this sandwich, inspired by Dive!'s popular Brick Oven Mushroom and Turkey Cheese Sub, you will likely not have the luxury of a brick oven to roast the mushrooms, but I've found the recipe is just as tasty as the real thing with sautéed mushrooms. It's important that you find the freshest bread your market has available, and if possible, get the turkey sliced for you at a full-service deli counter. A sandwich is only as good and as fresh as its ingredients, so try to find the best your market has to offer.

4 mushrooms, sliced (½ to ¾ cup)	6 ounces deli-sliced, roasted turkey breast
1 tablespoon butter	¼ cup White Cheddar Dipping Sauce (page 124)
Salt	1 7-inch baguette, sliced open
Pepper	2 ounces Swiss cheese, sliced

1. Preheat the oven to 450 degrees F.
2. Sauté the mushroom slices in the butter. Season with salt and pepper.

129

3. Heat the roasted turkey breast in a microwave oven or in another pan until warm.
4. Heat the White Cheddar Dipping Sauce until it is hot, if it's not hot already.

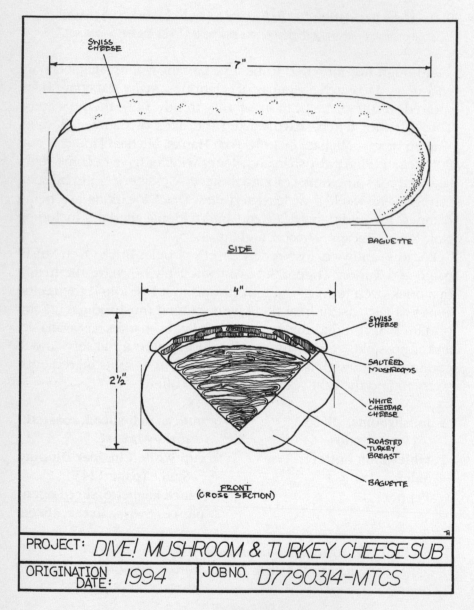

SWISS CHEESE

7"

SIDE

BAGUETTE

4"

SWISS CHEESE

SAUTÉED MUSHROOMS

2½"

WHITE CHEDDAR CHEESE

ROASTED TURKEY BREAST

BAGUETTE

FRONT
(CROSS SECTION)

PROJECT: DIVE! MUSHROOM & TURKEY CHEESE SUB

ORIGINATION DATE: 1994   JOB NO. D7790314-MTCS

5. Split the baguette without cutting all of the way through. Hinge the bread open and spread some of the cheese sauce on the faces of the bread.
6. Load the turkey breast into the sliced baguette. Salt and pepper it.
7. Pour the remaining cheese sauce over the turkey.
8. Spread the mushrooms over the cheese sauce.
9. Bake the open sandwich for 4 minutes. Put the Swiss cheese on top of the other ingredients and bake for 2 minutes more, or just until the cheese is melted. Slice the sandwich in half before serving.

✳ Dive! S'mores

Serves 2 to 4

Menu Description: "Graham crackers, milk chocolate and toasted marshmallows, streaked with chocolate sauce."

Large screens inside each Dive! display videos of underwater scenes filmed in the waters of Micronesia, Bermuda, San Salvador, and Florida. Diners eat gourmet submarine sandwiches as giant sea turtles and sharks swim by coral reefs and underwater caves. When the alarm sounds and lights flash, it's time for the restaurant to take its simulated hourly dive. Video in the portholes and on the giant projection screens changes to comedy footage from vintage movies and clips of unlikely locales for a huge submarine such as a backyard swimming pool.

Along with the two dozen or so gourmet sandwiches and other tasty entrees, Dive! features a delectable selection of desserts. One of them is Dive! S'mores, a creation inspired by the traditional treat that's prepared around campfires with marshmallows toasted on sticks. This version assembled with graham crackers, chocolate bars, and marshmallows is broiled in a hot oven just long enough to brown the tops of the marshmallows. If you've got a craving for S'mores and are nowhere near a campfire and/or don't have sticks, here's your quick fix.

2 **whole graham crackers (4 sections, not separated)**
2 **1½-ounce Hershey milk chocolate bars**

16 **large marshmallows**
2 **tablespoons Hershey's chocolate syrup, in squirt bottle**

1. Preheat the broiler. Arrange the graham crackers side by side on an oven-safe plate (such as ceramic). You can also use a baking sheet.
2. Stack the milk chocolate bars side by side on top of the graham crackers.

3. Arrange the marshmallows on the chocolate in 4 rows— 4 across, 4 down.
4. Broil the dessert on the middle rack for 1 to 3 minutes or until the marshmallows turn light brown on top.

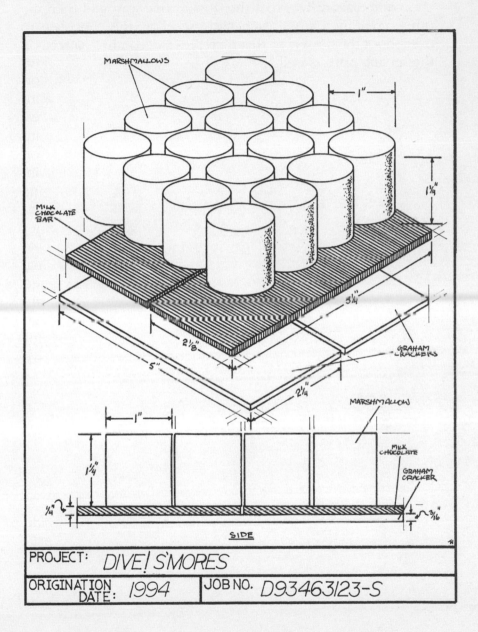

MARSHMALLOWS

MILK CHOCOLATE BAR

1"

1¼"

5¼"

2⅛"

5"

2¼"

GRAHAM CRACKERS

MARSHMALLOW

MILK CHOCOLATE

GRAHAM CRACKER

1"

1¼"

¼"

3/16"

SIDE

PROJECT: *DIVE! S'MORES*

ORIGINATION DATE: *1994*   JOB NO. *D93463123-S*

5. Remove the dessert from the oven. If you used a baking sheet, carefully slide the dessert onto a serving plate. With the squirt bottle, immediately drizzle the chocolate syrup over the marshmallows in a sweeping back-and-forth motion. Drizzle the chocolate diagonally across the dessert one way, and then the other, creating a cross-hatch pattern. Allow the chocolate to over-shoot the dessert so that it creates a decorative pattern on the serving plate as well.

✳ Hard Rock Cafe
Filet Steak Sandwich

Serves 2 as an entree

Menu Description: "Filet mignon grilled to perfection, sliced thin, with shredded lettuce, tomato and spicy mustard. Served on a sourdough French roll with fries and a salad."

When the first Hard Rock Cafe opened in 1971 on Old Park Lane in London, England, not one guitar or gold record decorated the walls. The burger joint was the inspiration of two Americans, Peter Morton and Isaac Tigrett, who couldn't find a decent American-style hamburger anywhere in London and decided to do something about it. The restaurant soon became famous only for its food, until along came Eric Clapton, who donated his guitar as a joke. Up on the wall it went. Not wanting to be outdone, Pete Townsend of The Who soon offered up a guitar of his own to be hung on the wall next to Clapton's with a note: "Mine's as good as his." That started a wave of donations from rock and rollers through the decades; and thus was born the world's first theme restaurant. Soon more Hard Rock Cafes were opening around the world, with the first one in America opening in Los Angeles in 1982. After that came New York City, San Francisco, Chicago, Houston, New Orleans, Maui, Las Vegas, Aspen, Newport Beach, and many more—a total of 58 so far. The success of the Hard Rock Cafe spawned a trend which now includes other restaurants built around themes ranging from movies to fashion to motorcycles to blues.

Here is an easy-to-make sandwich that features a tender, sliced filet mignon. It's a clone of one of the Hard Rock's more popular recent additions to the menu. This recipe suggests another way you can serve those filet mignons you've been saving in the freezer.

2 6- to 8-ounce filet mignon steaks	3 tablespoons mayonnaise
Salt and pepper	3 tablespoons spicy mustard
2 sourdough French rolls	6 slices tomato
	1 cup shredded iceberg lettuce

135

1. Preheat the barbecue or stovetop grill.
2. Since most filets are usually cut pretty thick (1 inch or more) you will want to slice your filets through the middle before grilling, making four thinner filets that are around ½ inch each.

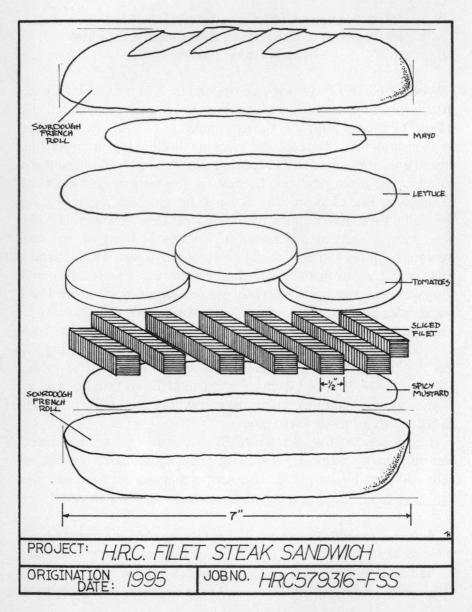

SOURDOUGH FRENCH ROLL

MAYO

LETTUCE

TOMATOES

SLICED FILET

←½"→

SPICY MUSTARD

SOURDOUGH FRENCH ROLL

|←——— 7" ———→|

PROJECT: *H.R.C. FILET STEAK SANDWICH*

ORIGINATION DATE: *1995*

JOB NO. *HRC579316-FSS*

3. Cook your filets over a hot grill for 2 to 4 minutes per side or until cooked to your preference. Be sure to salt and pepper both sides of each filet.
4. As the meat cooks, prepare your rolls by slicing them into top and bottom halves.
5. Spread the mayonnaise on the face of each top half.
6. Spread the mustard onto the face of each bottom half.
7. When the filets are done, slice them into ½-inch-thick strips.
8. Arrange the sliced filets evenly over the mustard on each bottom roll.
9. Place the tomato slices over the filets.
10. Put the shredded lettuce on top of the tomatoes.
11. Place the top buns on the lettuce and slice the sandwiches diagonally into two even halves. Hold each sandwich half together with toothpicks to serve.

✳ Hard Rock Cafe
Grilled Vegetable Sandwich

Serves 2 as an entree

Menu Description: "Grilled eggplant, zucchini, summer squash,
and roasted red peppers. Served on a sourdough French roll with
your choice of fries or watermelon."

Pop artist Andy Warhol called Hard Rock Cafe the "Smithsonian of Rock and Roll." In fact, the Hard Rock Cafe chain owns more artifacts of rock history than anyone in the world—somewhere around 30,000 in all. The chain has been collecting the artifacts, which decorate each of the 58 Hard Rock Cafes, for more than two decades. Because of this, some of the memorabilia you see in the restaurants, especially the older ones, were donated from artists even before they were famous.

As the chain grew larger over the years, cofounders Peter Morton and Isaac Tigrett grew tired of their business relationship. The company was eventually divided, with Isaac operating foreign Hard Rocks, and Peter taking over the stateside cafes. In 1988, Isaac sold his shares to Britain's Rank Organization and then partnered with actor Dan Aykroyd to open the House of Blues chain. In 1996, just a week before the Hard Rock celebrated its 25th anniversary, Peter sold his shares to Rank as well (for $410 million in cash!), consolidating the chain once again.

If you don't eat meat, or even if you do, you'll find this grilled vegetable sandwich makes a great meal in itself for lunch or dinner. I'm not usually one to go for strictly vegetarian sandwiches, but when I first tried this one I was surprised at how good it was. Now I veg out with this sandwich regularly. Hopefully you will too.

6 tablespoons mayonnaise	1 red bell pepper
½ teaspoon chopped fresh parsley	1 small zucchini
Pinch dried oregano	1 yellow summer squash
Salt	¼ eggplant
	¼ cup olive oil

2 sourdough French
   rolls
1 tablespoon freshly
   grated Parmesan
   cheese

6 to 8 separated onion ring
   slices (2 whole slices)
3 to 4 slices tomato
   (1 medium tomato)
2 leaves red leaf lettuce

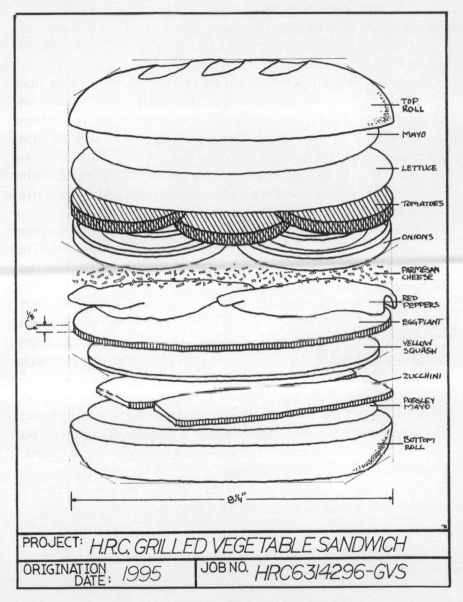

PROJECT: *H.R.C. GRILLED VEGETABLE SANDWICH*

ORIGINATION DATE: *1995*   JOB NO. *HRC6314296-GVS*

139

1. Preheat the barbecue or stovetop grill.
2. To prepare a spread, put 3 tablespoons of the mayo into a small bowl and add the parsley, oregano and a pinch of salt. Set this and the remaining mayonnaise aside until you're ready to make the sandwich.
3. Prepare the bell pepper by cutting it into quarters and seeding it. Brush the entire surface of the pepper with olive oil.
4. Slice the zucchini, squash, and eggplant into lengthwise slices no more than ⅛ to ¼ inch thick. Brush these slices with oil as well.
5. Cook the red pepper on a hot grill for 2 or 3 minutes. At that point add the remaining vegetables to the grill and cook everything for 4 to 5 more minutes or until all the vegetables are tender. Be sure to salt the vegetables and, of course, turn them halfway through the cooking time.
6. When the veggies are tender and begin to char, remove them from the grill and prepare each sandwich by first cutting the French rolls in half lengthwise through the middle.
7. Spread the parsley-mayonnaise over the face of the bottom halves.
8. Arrange the zucchini onto the rolls.
9. Stack the yellow squash next.
10. Eggplant goes on top of that.
11. Peel the skin off the red peppers, then stack the peppers on the eggplant.
12. Divide the Parmesan cheese and sprinkle it over the peppers.
13. Arrange the onions on the peppers.
14. Tomato slices go on the onions.
15. Tear the red lettuce leaves so that they fit on the tomatoes.
16. Divide the remaining 3 tablespoons of mayonnaise and spread it on the face of the top rolls and stack the rolls on the lettuce to finish off your sandwiches.
17. Cut the sandwiches diagonally through the middle and pierce each half with a toothpick before serving.

✳ Hard Rock Cafe Famous Baby Rock Watermelon Ribs

Serves 2 to 4 as an entree

Menu Description: "Texas style ribs basted in our special watermelon B.B.Q. sauce, grilled and served with fries and a green salad."

The collection of rock and roll memorabilia is different in each Hard Rock Cafe. You may find artifacts that come from recording stars of the fifties, like Elvis Presley and Fats Domino, to more contemporary artists such as Prince, Pearl Jam, and Nirvana. Usually there are several gold and platinum records donated from artists, sequined stage costumes, and famous guitars, some even left in a smashed condition as they were donated straight from a performance. The Hard Rock also collects movie memorabilia, such as Tom Cruise's pilot helmet from the movie *Top Gun* and the Indiana Jones jacket from *Raiders of the Lost Ark*.

In 1995, Hard rock cofounder Peter Morton opened the world's first rock-and-roll hotel, The Hard Rock Hotel and Casino, in Las Vegas. Peter now operates the hotel and his swank restaurant Morton's in Hollywood, California—the famous location of many a celebrity power meal over the years.

I thought these ribs with a barbecue sauce made from watermelon rind had a unique and memorable flavor begging to be duplicated at your next power meal. The sauce is sweet and slightly tangy, and the ribs are so tender they melt in your mouth. It's the slow-cooking process that makes them that way. Throwing them on the grill at the last minute is not meant to cook them so much as it is to add the smoky flavor and slight charring that good ribs require. If possible, make the watermelon barbecue sauce a day ahead so the ribs can marinate in it overnight. If you don't have time for that, at least marinate the ribs for a couple of hours.

141

**Watermelon rind from
  about ½ of a small
  watermelon**
1 cup dark corn syrup
½ cup water
¼ cup tomato ketchup

¼ cup distilled vinegar
**¾ teaspoon crushed red
  pepper flakes**
½ teaspoon liquid smoke
¼ teaspoon black pepper
4 pounds baby back ribs

1. For the puréed watermelon rind, you want to cut off the green skin and about half an inch of the hard white part, keeping the part of the watermelon that is lighter red to white. This is the tender part of the rind. Try to stay away from the harder, white rind just inside the green skin. Put the rind into a food processor and purée for only about 10 seconds. Strain the liquid from the pulp and use 1 cup of pulp, measured after straining.
2. Combine the watermelon pulp with the remaining ingredients for the sauce in a medium saucepan over high heat. Bring the mixture to a boil, then reduce the heat and simmer, covered, for about 1 hour or until it's as thick as you like it.
3. Cut racks of ribs into plate-size portions of about 6 or 7 rib bones each. Brush the ribs with the barbecue sauce and wrap each rack individually in aluminum foil. Be sure to save some sauce for later. Let the ribs marinate in the refrigerator for a couple of hours at least. (Overnight is best.)
4. Preheat the oven to 300 degrees F. To cook the ribs, set them with the seam of the foil facing up, into the oven. Bake for 2 to 2½ hours or until the rib meat has pulled back from the cut end of the bones by about ½ inch. They should be very tender.
5. Remove the ribs from the foil and brush on some additional sauce. Grill the ribs on a hot barbecue for 2 to 4 minutes per side or until you see several spots of charred sauce. Be sure to watch the ribs so that they do not burn. Serve with leftover sauce on the side.

✳ Hard Rock Cafe
Orange Freeze

Serves 1 as dessert or beverage

Menu Description: "Fresh squeezed O.J. and orange sherbet."

The Hard Rock Cafe chain has been committed to a "Save the Planet" campaign for some time now. The chain recycles all of the glass bottles, paper, and cardboard boxes, and uses no polystyrene. Water in the restaurant is only served on request. At the restaurants in Los Angeles and Newport Beach electronic tote boards have been erected to "tick away by the second the acres of remaining rainforest on the planet while also displaying the world's population count as it continues to explode, reminding us all to be conscious of our decreasing natural resources." In addition, any leftover food is donated to local charities that feed the homeless. That's cool, eh?

You'll find the Orange Freeze is pretty cool also, especially on a hot summer day. This refreshing dessert item at the Hard Rock is easy to duplicate at home with just a few ingredients and a couple minutes in front of a blender.

2 **cups orange sherbet or**   ¼ **cup milk**
    sorbet   1 **sprig of fresh spearmint**
1 **cup fresh squeezed orange**
    juice

1. Put the sherbet, juice, and milk in a blender and blend for 15 seconds or just until all the sherbet is smooth. You may have to stop the blender and stir the sherbet up a bit to help it combine.
2. Pour the orange freeze into a tall, chilled glass. Place a sprig of fresh spearmint in the top and serve immediately.

Tidbits

This is also good with a little whipped cream on top.

✳ Hooters
Buffalo Chicken Wings

Serves 3 to 5 as an appetizer

Menu Description: "Nearly world famous. Often imitated, hardly ever duplicated."

"Hooters is to chicken wings what McDonald's is to hamburgers," claims promotional material from the company. True, the six fun-loving midwestern businessmen who started Hooters in Clearwater, Florida, on April Fool's Day in 1983 chose a classic recipe for chicken wings as their feature item. But while some might say it's the Buffalo Wings that are their favorite feature of Hooters, others say it's the restaurant chain's trademark Hooters girls—waitresses casually attired in bright orange short-shorts and skin-tight T-shirts. Apparently it's a combination that works.

Today there are nearly 200 Hooters across the United States serving more than 150 tons of chicken wings every week. I've tasted lots of chicken wings, and I think these are some of the best wings served in any restaurant chain today. The original dish can be ordered in 10-, 20- or 50-piece servings; or if you want to splurge, there's the "Gourmet Chicken Wing Dinner" featuring 20 wings and a bottle of Dom Perignon champagne, for only $125. To further enhance the Hooters experience when you serve these messy wings, throw a whole roll of paper towels on the table, rather than napkins, as they do in the restaurants.

Vegetable oil for frying	Dash garlic powder
¼ cup butter	½ cup all-purpose flour
¼ cup Crystal Louisiana Hot Sauce or Frank's Red Hot Cayenne Sauce	¼ teaspoon paprika
	¼ teaspoon cayenne pepper
	¼ teaspoon salt
Dash ground pepper	10 chicken wing pieces

On the Side

Bleu cheese dressing	Celery sticks

1. Heat oil in a deep fryer to 375 degrees F. You want just enough oil to cover the wings entirely—an inch or so deep at least.
2. Combine the butter, hot sauce, ground pepper, and garlic powder in a small saucepan over low heat. Heat until the butter is melted and the ingredients are well-blended.

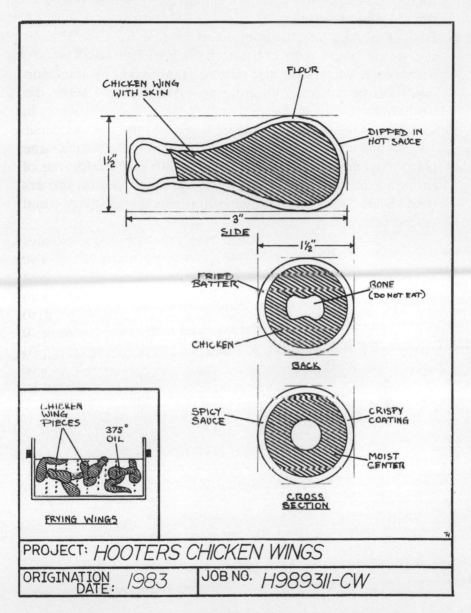

3. Combine the flour, paprika, cayenne pepper, and salt in a small bowl.
4. If the wings are frozen, be sure to defrost and dry them. Put the wings into a large bowl and sprinkle the flour mixture over them, coating each wing evenly. Put the wings in the refrigerator for 60 to 90 minutes. (This will help the breading to stick to the wings when fried.)
5. Put all the wings into the hot oil and fry them for 10 to 15 minutes or until some parts of the wings begin to turn dark brown.
6. Remove the wings from the oil to a paper towel to drain. But don't let them sit too long, because you want to serve the wings hot.
7. Quickly put the wings into a large bowl. Add the hot sauce and stir, coating all of the wings evenly. You could also use a large plastic container (such as Tupperware) with a lid for this. Put all the wings inside the container, add the sauce, put on the lid, then shake. Serve with bleu cheese dressing and celery sticks on the side.

✳ Hooters Buffalo Shrimp

Serves 3 to 4 as an appetizer

Menu Description: "It don't get no batter than this."

With the double-entendre name and female servers (many of whom, off-duty, are models), Hooters has become a company with critics. Several years ago a group of Hooters Girls in Minneapolis sued the company on grounds of sexual harassment, saying that the uniforms featuring shorts and tight T-shirts or tank tops were demeaning. Ultimately, the women dropped the suit. But more recently, the Equal Employment Opportunity Commission ordered the company to hire men on the foodservice staff. Hooters countered with a sarcastic million-dollar advertising campaign featuring a mustachioed man named "Vince" dressed in Hooters Girl getup. Once again, that suit was dropped.

Vice president of marketing Mike McNeil told *Nation's Restaurant News*, "Hooters Girls are actually wearing more clothing than what most women wear at the gym or the beach. It's part of the concept. I don't think the world would be a better place if we had guys be Hooters Girls." You may agree or disagree, but the fact is that Hooters is currently the country's thirteenth largest dinner house chain and one of the fastest growing, with an increasing number of diners discovering Buffalo Shrimp, a delicious spin-off of Buffalo Chicken Wings.

Vegetable oil for frying	Dash garlic powder
¼ cup butter	⅛ teaspoon paprika
¼ cup Crystal Louisiana Hot	12 uncooked large shrimp
Sauce or Frank's Red Hot	1 egg, beaten
Cayenne Sauce	½ cup milk
Dash ground pepper	1 cup all-purpose flour

On the Side

Lemon wedges

1. Heat oil in a deep fryer to 375 degrees F. You want the oil deep enough to cover the shrimp completely.
2. Combine the butter, hot sauce, ground pepper, garlic powder, and paprika in a small saucepan over low heat. Heat until the butter is melted and the ingredients are well blended.

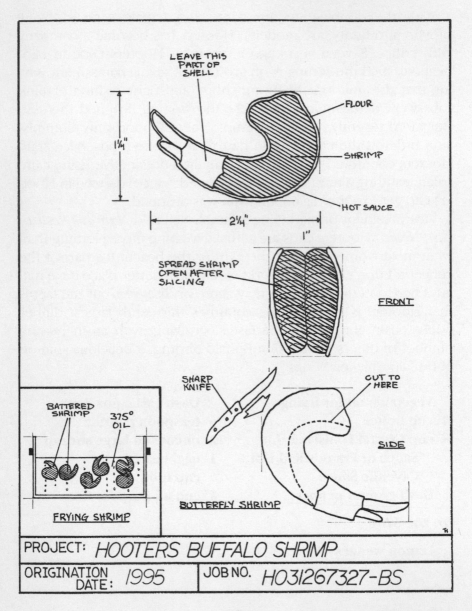

LEAVE THIS PART OF SHELL

FLOUR

SHRIMP

HOT SAUCE

1¼"

2¼"

1"

SPREAD SHRIMP OPEN AFTER SLICING

FRONT

SHARP KNIFE

CUT TO HERE

SIDE

BATTERED SHRIMP

375° OIL

FRYING SHRIMP

BUTTERFLY SHRIMP

PROJECT: *HOOTERS BUFFALO SHRIMP*

ORIGINATION DATE: *1995*

JOB NO. *HO31267327-BS*

3. Prepare the shrimp by cutting off the entire shell, leaving only the last segment of the shell and the tailfins. Remove the vein from the back and clean the shrimp. Then, with a paring knife, cut a deeper slice where you removed the vein (down to the tail), so that you can fan the meat out. Be careful not to cut too deep. This will butterfly the shrimp.
4. Combine the egg with the milk in a small bowl. Put the flour into another bowl.
5. Dredge each shrimp in the milk mixture, then coat it with the flour. Make sure each shrimp is evenly coated. When you have coated all of the shrimp with flour, let them sit for about 10 minutes in the refrigerator before frying.
6. Fry the shrimp in the hot oil for 7 to 10 minutes or until the tip of each tail begins to turn dark brown. Remove the shrimp from the oil to paper towels briefly, to drain.
7. Quickly put the shrimp into a large bowl, add the hot sauce and stir, coating each shrimp evenly. You could also use a large plastic container with a lid for this. Put all the shrimp inside, add the sauce, put on the lid, then gently turn the container over a few times to coat all of the shrimp. Serve with wedges of lemon on the side.

✳ Hooters Pasta Salad

Serves 4 as a lunch or light dinner

Menu Description: *"Rotini, cukes, tomatoes, scallions and vinaigrette dressing on the side."*

On the back of each menu at this popular dinner house chain is the "Hooters Saga"—a tongue-in-cheek tale of the restaurant's origin. The story claims that the chain's founders, referred to as "the Hooters Six," were arrested shortly after opening the first Hooters restaurant "for impersonating restauranteurs (sic). There were no indictments," the story explains. "But the stigma lingers on."

Even though the "saga" claims the building for the first Hooters restaurant was originally going to be used as a "giant walk-in dumpster," each Hooters outlet is designed to look like a Florida beachhouse. And whether it's December or July, day or night, you'll notice the trademark multicolored Christmas lights are always on.

Since Hooters is more than just Buffalo wings and shrimp, I thought I'd include a clone for a newer item on the menu. You'll love the tasty tri-color pasta salad tossed with tomatoes, cucumbers, and green onion, and a delicious vinaigrette. Use this Top Secret version of the pink vinaigrette dressing on a variety of salads or sub sandwiches, or even as a marinade.

Vinaigrette Dressing

⅔ cup vegetable oil
⅓ cup red wine vinegar
1½ tablespoons sugar
1 tablespoon Grey Poupon Dijon mustard
2 teaspoons minced shallot
1 teaspoon lemon juice
½ teaspoon dried thyme

¼ teaspoon dried parsley flakes
¼ teaspoon garlic powder
⅛ teaspoon salt
⅛ teaspoon coarsely ground black pepper
⅛ teaspoon dried basil
⅛ teaspoon dried oregano
Dash onion powder

4 quarts water	1 large or 2 medium tomatoes
1 pound rainbow rotini or tri-color radiatore (red, green, and white colors)	1 green onion
	¼ cup minced cucumber
	Salt
	Green leaf lettuce
1 to 2 teaspoons vegetable oil	(optional, for garnish)

1. Make the dressing: Use an electric mixer to combine all of the dressing ingredients in a bowl. Mix on high speed for about a minute or so until the dressing becomes thick and creamy. Put the dressing in a sealed container and store it in the refrigerator until ready to toss with the chilled pasta.
2. Bring 4 quarts of water to a boil over high heat and add the pasta. Cook for 12 to 14 minutes, until tender, then drain it.
3. Spray the pasta with a gentle stream of cold water to help cool it off. Drizzle the oil over the cooling pasta to keep it from sticking together. Gently toss the pasta, then put it into a covered container and let it cool in the refrigerator for 30 minutes or so.
4. While the pasta is cooling down, prepare the vegetables: remove the seeds and soft pulp from the tomato(es) before dicing; use only the green part of the green onion (or scallions); and be sure to mince the cucumber into very small pieces.
5. When the pasta is no longer warm, add the diced tomato, green onion, and cucumber. Sprinkle salt over the pasta salad to taste and put it back in the refrigerator until well chilled.
6. When the pasta has chilled, spoon it onto plates and place the vinaigrette dressing on the side. For a cool garnish like that served in the restaurant, spread some leaves of green leaf lettuce onto each plate, then spoon the pasta onto the lettuce. You may also toss the salad with the dressing ahead of time rather than serving it on the side. But don't do this too far in advance or the pasta tends to soak up the dressing.

Tidbits

Although I didn't detect it in the original vinaigrette dressing for this pasta salad, for best flavor I recommend substituting ½ clove of minced or grated garlic into the blend, for the ¼ teaspoon of garlic powder.

151

✳ Houlihan's Houli Fruit Fizz

Serves 2

Menu Description: "Houlihan's own blend of Ocean Spray Cranberry Juice Cocktail, orange juice, pineapple juice and Sprite."

Restaurateurs Joseph Gilbert and John Robinson needed a name for the new restaurant they planned to open in the Country Club Plaza of Kansas City, Missouri. To make the job easy, they kept the name of the location's previous tenant—a clothing store called Houlihan's Men's Wear—and opened Houlihan's Old Place in 1972. This was at the time when T.G.I. Friday's was popularizing casual dining, so the concept was an instant hit. That early success led to more Houlihan's opening in other states, and another multi-million dollar chain was born.

The Houli Fruit Fizz is a simple blend of fruit juices and Sprite that can be served with a meal or enjoyed on its own. This drink is one of Houlihan's own classic, signature recipes.

1 12-ounce can cold Sprite   ¼ cup cold orange juice
½ cup cold pineapple juice   1 cup cold cranberry juice

Combine all of the ingredients in a pitcher and pour into two glasses over ice. Be sure all of the ingredients are cold when combined.

✳ Houlihan's 'Shrooms

Serves 2 to 3 as an appetizer

Menu Description: "Jumbo mushroom caps filled with herb and garlic cheese, lightly battered and fried. Served with zesty horseradish and mustard dip made with Grey Poupon."

In a March 1986 story which ran in the *Kansas City Times*, a feud erupted between Gilbert/Robinson, the parent company of Houlihan's restaurant at the time, and two guys building their own chain of bars called Mike Houlihan's. The president of the Houlihan's chain, Fred Hipp, said that at first Houlihan's didn't mind so much, asking kindly that the name not be used. But when Mike Heyer and John Houlihan opened a Mike Houlihan's in St. Louis only a few blocks away from an original Houlihan's restaurant, Fred saw no choice but to sue. Soon, residents with the surname Houlihan were writing to Fred urging him to drop the lawsuit. "You'll feel better, thirteen hundred Houlihans will feel better, and two stubborn Irishmen will have $50,000 to buy more Irish whiskey," said one letter.

Here's another Houlihan's classic recipe called 'Shrooms: cheese-filled, batter-fried mushrooms served piping hot. You have the choice of making the herb-flavored cheese filling from the recipe here, or if you're feeling especially lazy, you can buy a similar pre-made filling (check out the "Tidbits"). Be careful when you first bite into these puppies. Straight out of the fryer, the hot cheese filling can squirt from the center and inflict burning pain on your tongue and lips similar to that of molten lava. Believe me, I know.

Herb Cheese Filling

⅛ teaspoon dried summer savory
⅛ teaspoon garlic powder
⅛ teaspoon salt

6 to 8 large button mushrooms
1 cup unbleached flour
1½ teaspoons salt

Dash dried parsley flakes
Dash dried tarragon
Dash ground pepper
⅓ cup whipped cream cheese
½ teaspoon cayenne pepper
½ cup milk
Vegetable oil for frying

153

Dipping Sauce

½ cup mayonnaise
2 teaspoons Grey Poupon
  Dijon mustard
1 teaspoon white vinegar

2 teaspoons prepared
  horseradish
½ teaspoon sugar

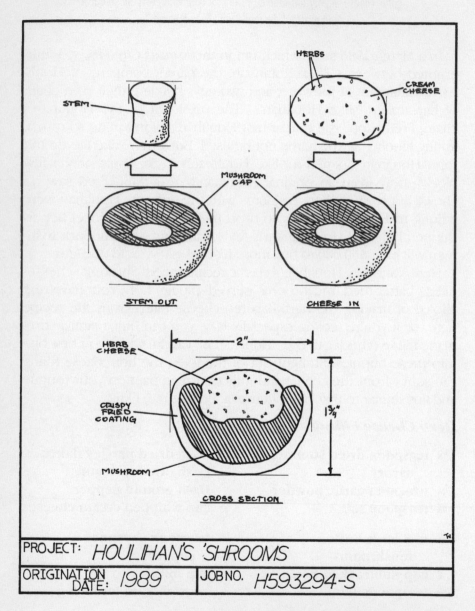

HERBS

CREAM CHEESE

STEM

MUSHROOM CAP

STEM OUT

CHEESE IN

HERB CHEESE

2"

CRISPY FRIED COATING

1¾"

MUSHROOM

CROSS SECTION

PROJECT: HOULIHAN'S 'SHROOMS

ORIGINATION DATE: 1989

JOB NO. H593294-S

1. Combine the savory, garlic powder, ⅛ teaspoon salt, parsley, tarragon, and pepper in a small bowl and use your fingers or the back of a spoon to crush the spices into much smaller pieces. If you have a mortar and pestle, use that. Just be sure you don't pulverize the spices into dust.
2. Combine the spice mixture with the cream cheese and let it sit for 10 to 15 minutes or longer so that the flavors integrate.
3. Clean the mushrooms and remove the stems, leaving only the caps.
4. When the cheese has rested, use a teaspoon to fill the mushroom caps with the herb cheese.
5. Combine the flour with 1½ teaspoons salt and the cayenne pepper in a small bowl.
6. Pour the milk into another small bowl.
7. Dip each mushroom first in the milk then into the flour mixture. Do this twice for each mushroom so that each one has been double-coated with flour.
8. Put the coated mushrooms into the freezer for at least 3 hours. This will keep the coating from falling off, and it will keep the cheese inside from expanding too fast and leaking out of the mushroom when frying.
9. Meanwhile, make the dipping sauce by combining all of the ingredients in a small bowl. Keep the sauce covered and chilled until you are ready to serve it.
10. When the mushrooms are frozen, heat the oil in a deep fryer or deep pot to 350 degrees F. Use enough oil to completely cover the mushrooms (at least a couple inches deep). Fry the mushrooms for 8 to 10 minutes or until the outside turns golden brown. Drain the mushrooms on a rack or paper towels. Let the mushrooms sit for a couple minutes before serving—they will be very hot inside. Serve with dipping sauce on the side.

Tidbits

If you're feeling lazy, rather than make your own cheese filling you can purchase one of the 4-ounce preblended herb cheeses made by Rondele or Alouette. They're usually found near the cream cheese in the supermarket.

You can also make a lighter version of this recipe by substituting a lower fat cream cheese. The preblended cheeses come in light versions as well.

✳ Houlihan's Smashed Potatoes

Serves 4 as a side dish

Here's a great way to make mashed potatoes, Houlihan's style. The Smashed Potatoes at the restaurant chain are considered one of Houlihan's specialty signature dishes. This à la carte dish is unique because of the added fresh onion, spices, and sour cream; and especially because of the finishing touch—some onion straws sprinkled on top. It's important when making your own version that you not entirely mash the potatoes, but instead leave a few small potato chunks for texture. Once you make homemade mashed potatoes this way, you'll never want to make them any other way.

4 medium or 2 large russet
    potatoes, peeled
½ cup milk
½ teaspoon salt
¼ teaspoon coarsely ground
    black pepper
1 tablespoon fresh minced
    onion

2 tablespoons sour cream
Dash garlic powder
¼ cup French's French
    Fried Onions
    (onion straws)

1. Slice the potatoes into 1-inch cubes and boil in 6 cups of salted water for 15 to 20 minutes or until soft and tender.
2. Drain off the water and use a fork or potato masher to mash the potatoes. Stop mashing when there are still some small chunks of potato left. It's the chunky consistency that makes these potatoes unique.
3. Immediately add the remaining ingredients, excluding the fried onions, to the pan and put it back over low heat. Reheat the potatoes for 5 minutes, stirring to mix in the other ingredients.
4. Serve the potatoes with a sprinkling of about 1 tablespoon of fried onions on top of each serving.

Tidbits

If you wish, you can make the onion straws yourself following the recipe on page 246.

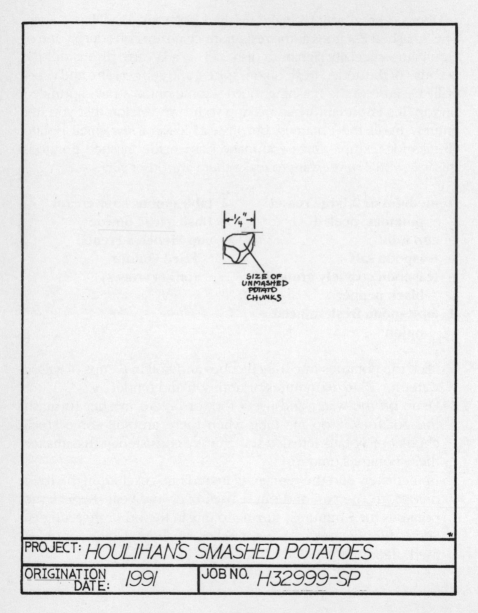

SIZE OF
UNMASHED
POTATO
CHUNKS

PROJECT: *HOULIHAN'S SMASHED POTATOES*

| ORIGINATION DATE: *1991* | JOB NO. *H32999-SP* |

✳ International House of Pancakes French Toast

Serves 2 (can be doubled)

Menu Description: "Six triangular slices with powdered sugar."

Now in its 38th year, IHOP has become one of the recognized leaders for breakfast dining, serving up thousands of omelettes, waffles, blintzes, and pancakes each and every day.

Among the popular morning meals is IHOP's classic French toast. You'll notice the addition of a little bit of flour to the batter to make this version of French toast more like the dish you get at the restaurant. The flour helps to create a thicker coating on the bread, almost like a tender crepe on the surface, keeping the bread from becoming too soggy.

2 **eggs**	⅛ **teaspoon salt**
½ **cup milk**	3 **teaspoons butter**
1 **teaspoon vanilla**	6 **slices thick-sliced French**
3 **tablespoons all-purpose**	**bread**
flour	1 **tablespoon powdered sugar**

On the Side

Butter   **Pancake syrup**

1. Beat the eggs in a large shallow bowl.
2. Add the milk, vanilla, flour, and salt to the eggs. Beat the mixture with an electric mixer. Be sure all the flour is well combined.
3. Heat a large skillet over medium heat. When the surface is hot, add about a teaspoon of butter.
4. Dip the bread, a slice at a time, into the batter, being sure to coat each side well. Drop the bread into the hot pan (as many as will fit at one time) and cook for 2 to 3 minutes per side or until the surface is golden brown. Repeat with the remaining pieces of bread.
5. Cut each piece of toast in half diagonally. Arrange six halves

159

of the toast on two plates by neatly overlapping the slices. Sprinkle about ½ tablespoon of powdered sugar over the tops of the toast slices on each plate. Serve with butter and syrup on the side.

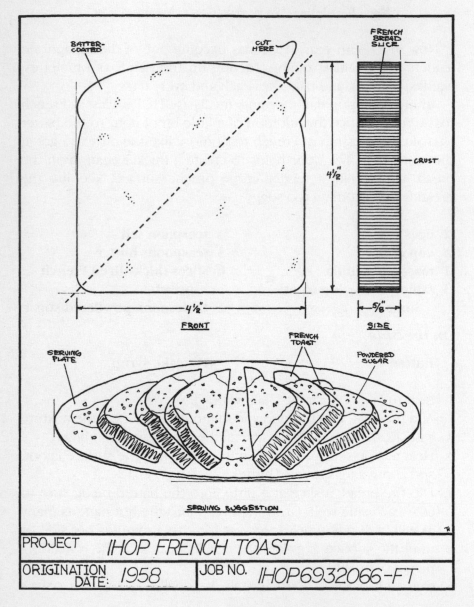

BATTER-COATED

CUT HERE

FRENCH BREAD SLICE

CRUST

4½"

4½"

⅝"

FRONT

SIDE

SERVING PLATE

FRENCH TOAST

POWDERED SUGAR

SERVING SUGGESTION

PROJECT	*IHOP FRENCH TOAST*	
ORIGINATION DATE: *1958*	JOB NO.	*IHOP6932066-FT*

✳ International House of Pancakes Cheese Blintz

Serves 3 to 4 (10 to 12 blintzes)

Menu Description: "Crepe-style pancakes filled with a blend of cheeses with strawberry preserves and sour cream."

Detroit's mayoral candidate Sharon McPhail and Detroit schools superintendent David Snead often dined in the city's hottest spot for power breakfasts—the local IHOP. Perhaps it was that first little something in common that eventually led to the two exchanging vows in front of 1,800 guests in a 1995 wedding ceremony. It was dubbed Detroit's "wedding of the year." That particular IHOP, which just happens to be owned by singer Anita Baker's husband, Walter Bridgforth, has seen a 200 percent jump in business.

You'll enjoy this simple recipe for crepes, which, when filled with cheese, become delicious blintzes. The restaurant uses a type of cheese that is similar to soft farmer's cheese, but you can make this with cream cheese, or even with yogurt that has been strained to make it thicker. Any way you decide to go, you're in for a treat.

Crepes

1½ cups all-purpose flour	2 eggs
2 cups milk	½ teaspoon vanilla
3 tablespoons butter, melted	½ teaspoon baking powder
	½ teaspoon salt
2 tablespoons granulated sugar	
	Butter (for pan)

Filling

1 cup cottage cheese	¼ cup powdered sugar
1 cup soft farmer cheese or softened cream cheese (see Tidbits)	¼ teaspoon vanilla

161

On the Side

Sour cream   **Powdered sugar**
Strawberry preserves

1. Use an electric mixer to blend together all the crepe ingredients except the butter for the pan in a large bowl. Blend just until smooth. The batter will be very thin.
2. Combine the filling ingredients in a medium bowl and mix by hand. Keep the filling nearby.
3. Preheat a 10-inch frying pan over medium heat. (This size pan tapers to about 8 inches at the bottom.) When the pan is hot, add about ½ teaspoon of butter.
4. When the butter has melted, pour ⅓ cup of batter into the pan. Swirl the batter so that it entirely coats the bottom of the pan. Cook for 1½ to 2 minutes or until golden brown on one side.
5. Use a spatula to lift an edge of the crepe. Grab it with your finger, slip the spatula underneath, and quickly flip it over. Cook for another 1½ minutes or until a bit lighter shade of brown than the first side, then slide it out of the pan. Repeat with the rest of the batter and stack the finished crepes on top of each other to keep them warm.
6. Heat the cheese filling in the microwave for 1 to 2 minutes or until it is hot.
7. When ready to fill the crepes, place each crepe, dark side down, on a plate. Pour 2 to 3 tablespoons of cheese filling across the center of the crepe. Fold the sides in and turn the entire blintz over (to hide the seam) onto a serving plate. You can use a knife to cut the rounded ends off the blintzes if you like. Repeat with the remaining blintzes.
8. Serve 2 to 3 blintzes on a plate with a dollop of sour cream and 2 dollops of strawberry preserves carefully arranged on the plate next to the blintzes. Sprinkle the blintzes with powdered sugar.

Tidbits

If you would like to make this recipe with a lowfat or nonfat filling, replace the cream cheese or farmer's cheese with strained yogurt—a yogurt solid that is thick like cheese. To make it, pour a cup of lowfat or nonfat yogurt into a coffee filter placed inside a strainer. Put the strainer over a bowl and into the refrigerator for 4 to 5 hours so that all of the liquid whey strains out of the yogurt. What you have left in the strainer is a thick, nutritious yogurt cheese that can be used in place of cream cheese or sour cream in this recipe and many others.

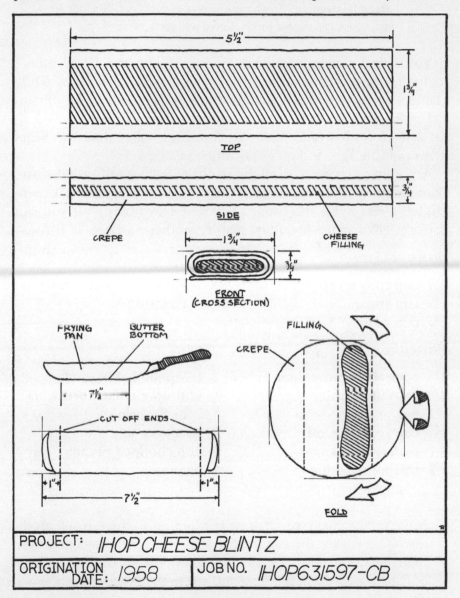

163

✳ International House of Pancakes Banana Nut Pancakes

Serves 3 to 4

Menu Description: *"Four banana-flavored pancakes garnished with fresh banana and chopped pecans. Served with banana-flavored syrup."*

You'll find sixteen varieties of pancakes on the IHOP menu, including one of the newest flavors: pumpkin pancakes. IHOP claims to sell over 400,000 pancakes each day. That's a lot of pancakes. So many, in fact, that if all of those flapjacks were served up on one plate, it would make a giant stack taller than the Sears Tower in Chicago. And probably much tastier.

According to servers, of all the pancake flavors and varieties, the Banana Nut Pancakes are one of the most often requested. I've included a recipe for the banana-flavored syrup here, but you can use any flavor syrup, including maple, on these babies.

Banana Syrup

½ cup corn syrup
½ cup sugar
½ cup water

¼ teaspoon banana extract or flavoring

Pancakes

1¼ cups all-purpose flour
1½ cups buttermilk
1 egg
¼ cup vegetable oil
2 tablespoons sugar
1 teaspoon baking powder

1 teaspoon baking soda
½ tablespoon banana extract or flavoring
¼ teaspoon salt
⅔ cup chopped pecans
1 banana

1. Make the banana syrup first by combining all the syrup ingredients—except for the banana extract—in a small saucepan over high heat, stirring occasionally. When the mixture begins to boil, remove it from the heat and stir in the banana extract.

2. In a large bowl, combine all the ingredients for the pancakes except the pecans and the banana. Use an electric mixer to blend until smooth.

3. Heat a large frying pan or griddle over medium heat, and coat it with butter or nonstick cooking spray when hot.

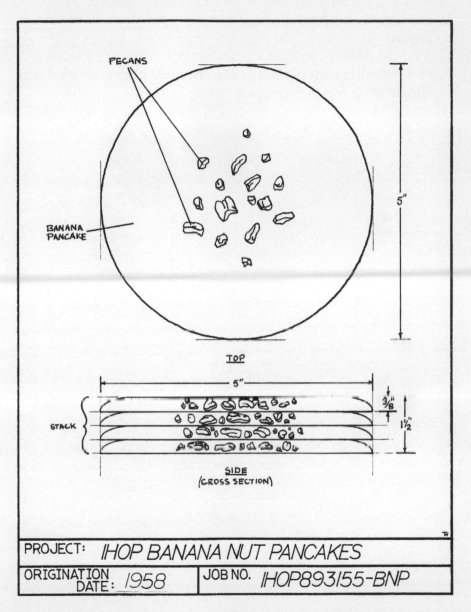

PECANS

BANANA
PANCAKE

5"

TOP

STACK

5"

3/8"

1½"

SIDE
(CROSS SECTION)

PROJECT: *IHOP BANANA NUT PANCAKES*

ORIGINATION DATE: *1958*

JOB NO. *IHOP893155-BNP*

4. Pour ¼-cup dollops of batter into the pan. Realize the batter will spread out to about 4 inches across, so leave enough room if you are cooking more than one at a time. Granted, some pans may only hold one or two at a time. Sprinkle about ½ tablespoon pecans into the center of each pancake immediately after you pour the batter so that the nuts are "cooked in."
5. Cook the pancakes for 1 to 2 minutes per side or until golden brown.
6. Slice the banana, divide it up, and serve it on top of a stack of 3 to 4 pancakes with the remaining chopped pecans divided and sprinkled on top of each stack.

✳ International House of Pancakes Fajita Omelette

Serves 2

Menu Description: "Seasoned chicken or beef with onions, diced green peppers, cheese, and chile salsa."

Pancakes are obviously the signature entree, but IHOP serves a variety of breakfast selections—more than 65 items! Along with a cup of coffee from the trademarked "Never Empty Coffee Pot," diners can choose from about a dozen different omelette selections including the Santa Fe Omelette, International Omelette, Chorizo and Cheese Omelette, and the delicious Fajita Omelette.

In my version of the original favorite, you can use either chicken or beef.

1 boneless, skinless chicken breast half *or* 6-ounce flank steak	¼ medium Spanish onion, diced (about ½ cup)
½ teaspoon vegetable oil	1 small tomato, diced (about ½ cup)
½ teaspoon lime juice	2 teaspoons butter
¼ teaspoon chili powder	5 large eggs, beaten
⅛ teaspoon salt	1 cup shredded Cheddar cheese
⅛ teaspoon cumin	
Dash garlic powder	⅓ cup salsa
Dash black pepper	2 tablespoons sour cream
½ green bell pepper, diced (about ½ cup)	

1. Pound the chicken breast or flank steak between sheets of plastic wrap until about ¼ inch thick, then cut the meat into bite-size pieces.
2. Pour the oil into a medium skillet over high heat. Add the meat and sauté it for a couple of minutes until it starts to brown.
3. Add the lime juice to the meat. Blend the spices together in a

167

small bowl, then add this mixture to the meat. Mix well until blended in.
4. Add the pepper and onion to the meat and simmer for 5 to 10 minutes over medium heat or until the veggies begin to turn brown. Add the tomato and cook another 2 minutes.

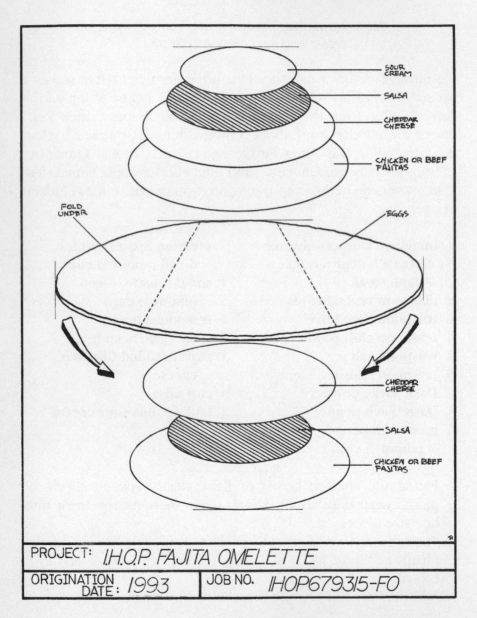

PROJECT: I.H.O.P. FAJITA OMELETTE

ORIGINATION DATE: 1993   JOB NO. IHOP679315-FO

5. Set a large skillet over medium heat. Add 1 teaspoon of butter to the pan.
6. When the butter has melted, add half of the beaten eggs to the pan and swirl to coat the entire bottom of the pan.
7. Cook the eggs for a minute or so or until the top surface is beginning to get firm. Be sure the bottom is not getting too brown before the top cooks. If you notice this happening, turn down the heat.
8. Sprinkle about ¼ cup of cheese down the center of the eggs.
9. Spoon a heaping tablespoon of salsa over the cheese.
10. Spoon one-fourth of the meat and vegetables onto the salsa.
11. Fold the edges over the center of the omelette and let it cook for another minute or so.
12. Carefully flip the omelette over in the pan with the seam side down. Let it cook for another minute or two, then slide it out onto a serving plate. Keep this omelette hot in a slow oven while you prepare the other one.
13. When both omelettes are done, spoon the remaining meat and vegetables over each of the omelettes.
14. Sprinkle a couple tablespoons of cheese over the other topping.
15. Add 2 tablespoons of salsa.
16. Then add a 1-tablespoon dollop of sour cream to the salsa on the middle of the omelette.

✳ Lone Star
Steakhouse & Saloon
Amarillo Cheese Fries

Serves 4 to 6 as an appetizer or snack

Menu Description: *"Lone Star fries smothered in Monterey Jack and Cheddar cheese, topped with bacon and served with ranch dressing."*

Growth by this newcomer to the steakhouse segment has been phenomenal. So far, there are over 160 Lone Stars across the country, most of them in the East and Midwest. There are even four in Australia. The company is the fastest growing steakhouse chain in the country, and if you don't have one near you yet, you probably will soon.

Amarillo Cheese Fries are made with thick-sliced unpeeled potatoes. The recipe here is created from scratch, using freshly sliced potatoes. But, if this is one of those days when you just don't feel up to slicing and frying some russets, you can also use a bag of frozen steak fries. Just be aware that those will likely be made from peeled potatoes, unlike the real thing that is served at the restaurant. I've also included a cool recipe for homemade ranch dressing to dip the fries in, if you decide you'd like to make yours from scratch.

3 unpeeled russet potatoes	1 cup shredded Monterey
4 to 6 cups vegetable oil for frying	Jack cheese
	3 slices bacon, cooked
1 cup shredded Cheddar cheese	⅓ cup ranch dressing

1. Slice the potatoes into wide rectangular slices. They should be about ¼ inch thick and ¾ inch wide. You should end up with around 12 to 15 slices per potato. Keep the potato slices immersed in water until they are ready to fry so that they don't turn brown.

2. Heat the oil in a deep fryer or deep pan to 350 degrees F. Dry the potato slices on paper towels and fry them for 1 minute in the hot oil. This is the blanching stage. Remove the potatoes from the oil and drain until they cool, about 10 minutes.
3. When the potato slices are cool, fry them for 5 more minutes or until they are a light golden brown. Drain.

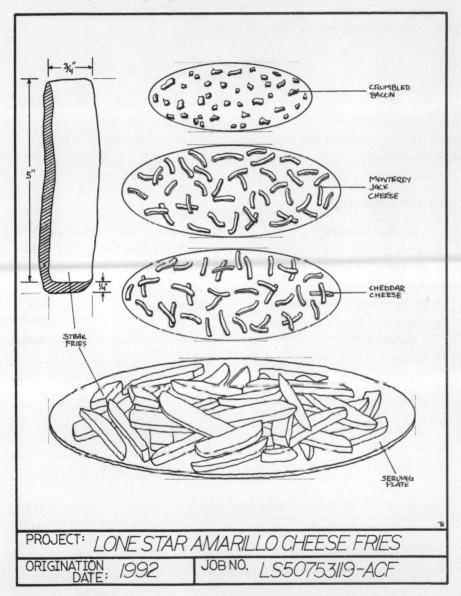

3/4"

5"

1/4"

CRUMBLED BACON

MONTEREY JACK CHEESE

CHEDDAR CHEESE

STEAK FRIES

SERVING PLATE

PROJECT: *LONE STAR AMARILLO CHEESE FRIES*

ORIGINATION DATE: *1992*

JOB NO. *LS5075319-ACF*

171

4. Preheat your oven to 375 degrees F, then arrange the fries on an oven-safe plate.
5. Sprinkle the Cheddar cheese over the fries.
6. Sprinkle the Monterey Jack cheese over the Cheddar.
7. Crumble the cooked bacon and sprinkle it over the cheese.
8. Bake the fries in the oven for 5 minutes or until the cheese has melted. Serve hot with bottled ranch dressing or make your own with the recipe offered here.

Tidbits

You can also make this recipe using a 32-ounce bag of store-bought frozen steak fries. Just cook them following the directions on the bag, adding the toppings in the last 5 minutes of baking.

If you want to make your own ranch dressing for dipping instead of buying it at the store, here is a good recipe that I came up with:

Ranch Dressing

¼ cup mayonnaise
1 tablespoon buttermilk
½ teaspoon sugar
¼ teaspoon vinegar
¼ teaspoon garlic powder
¼ teaspoon finely chopped
   fresh dill

¼ teaspoon finely chopped
   fresh parsley
⅛ teaspoon onion powder
Dash salt
Dash paprika

Combine all of the ingredients in a small bowl and let them chill for an hour or two.

✷ Lone Star Steakhouse & Saloon Black Bean Soup

Serves 4 as an appetizer, 2 as an entree

This restaurant boasts a unique "Texas roadhouse" ambiance. When you walk into any Lone Star restaurant, the first thing you'll notice is the crackling of peanut shells beneath your feet. When you're seated you get your own free bucket of peanuts to munch on, and you just flip the shells onto the wood plank floors. Western music plays over the speakers, and every hour or so the wait staff breaks into a funky little honky tonk line dance next to your table while the crunching peanut shells add a unique percussion element.

The spicy black bean soup is a popular item on the Lone Star menu. Here's a way to make a version of your own that can be served as an appetizer or as a meal in itself. It's great with a garnish of freshly diced red onion, jalapeños, and sour cream on top.

2 **15-ounce cans black beans**	1 **teaspoon cider or wine**
¼ **cup diced red onion**	**vinegar**
2 **teaspoons chopped pickled**	2 **cloves garlic, minced**
jalapeño slices ("nacho	¼ **teaspoon salt**
slices")	¼ **teaspoon cayenne pepper**
1 **teaspoon sugar**	½ **teaspoon chili powder**

Garnish

4 **teaspoons chopped red**	6 **to 8 jalapeño slices**
onion	1 **tablespoon sour cream**

1. Pour the canned beans along with the liquid into a medium saucepan. Add the remaining soup ingredients and mix.
2. Bring the soup to a boil, then reduce the heat to low and simmer, covered, for about 1 hour, adding water if necessary or until it's as thick as you like.

3. Serve each bowl of soup with a garnish of red onion, jalapeño slices, and sour cream arranged carefully in the center of the soup.

Tidbits

This soup is also very good with a bit of chopped fresh cilantro added to it while simmering and/or as a garnish. You may want to try some shredded Cheddar or Monterey Jack cheese on top as well.

✳ Lone Star Steakhouse & Saloon Texas Rice

Serves 2 as a side dish

The best selling menu items at the Lone Star Steakhouse & Saloon are the mesquite grilled steaks. The USDA choice-graded steaks are hand-cut fresh daily and displayed in a glass meat counter that is visible from the dining area of each restaurant. Customers are encouraged to view the meat for themselves and personally select the steak they wish to eat.

Even though much of the beef, chicken, and fish served at the restaurant is mesquite grilled, you may not have the equipment to cook your meat that way. Never fear, you can still have this popular and tasty side dish alongside another entree or steak cooked up any way you like. Rice this good goes with just about anything.

2 cups beef stock or canned beef broth	**1 tablespoon vegetable oil**
1 cup uncooked long grain parboiled or converted (*not* instant or quick) white rice	**⅓ cup diced white onion** **3 to 4 mushrooms, sliced** **½ cup frozen peas** **¼ teaspoon chili powder** **¼ teaspoon salt**

1. Bring the beef stock to a boil over high heat in a medium saucepan.
2. Add the rice to the stock, cover the pan, reduce heat to low, and simmer for 20 minutes.
3. When the rice has cooked for about 10 minutes, heat the oil in a skillet over medium heat.
4. When the oil is hot, add the onion and mushrooms to the pan and sauté for 5 minutes.
5. When the rice is done, pour it into the skillet with the mushrooms and onion. Turn the heat to medium/low and add the

frozen peas, chili powder, and salt to the rice. Heat the mixture, stirring often, for 3 to 4 minutes or until the peas are tender.

Tidbits

It's important that you use converted or parboiled rice for this recipe, and others that call for white rice. Sure, this type of rice may take longer to cook than instant rice, but all its nutrients and taste haven't been stripped out—which is exactly what happens in the process that creates the popular quick-cooking, 5-minute stuff. You don't need that junk. Converted rice is one of the best rices to use in cooking because it doesn't get too mushy or sticky, and the grains don't easily split open.

✳ Lone Star
Steakhouse & Saloon
Sweet Bourbon Salmon

Serves 2 as an entree

Menu Description: "Fresh salmon filet, marinated and mesquite grilled."

It is said that Americans eat an estimated 63 pounds of beef per capita, and we get a lot of it in chain restaurants. But for those of you who want something other than beef, Lone Star has additional selections including the Sweet Bourbon Salmon.

Don't worry if you can't mesquite grill your salmon, it's the sweet bourbon marinade that makes this dish so tasty. Not only is this marinade good on salmon, but on other fish and chicken as well. If you do happen to use a charcoal grill and have some mesquite smoking chips on hand, soak a handful of chips in water for a couple hours and then arrange them on the red-hot coals. This will give your salmon a taste even closer to the original.

Sweet Bourbon Marinade

¼ cup pineapple juice
2 tablespoons soy sauce
2 tablespoons brown sugar
1 teaspoon Kentucky bourbon

¼ teaspoon cracked black pepper
⅛ teaspoon garlic powder
½ cup vegetable oil

2 8-ounce salmon fillets

2 teaspoons snipped fresh chives

1. Combine the pineapple juice, soy sauce, brown sugar, bourbon, pepper and garlic powder in a medium bowl. Stir to dissolve the sugar. Add the oil.
2. Be sure all of the skin is removed from the salmon. Place the fillets in a shallow dish and pour the bourbon marinade over them, saving a little to brush on the fish as it cooks. Put a lid over the fish and refrigerate for at least an hour. A few hours is even better.

177

3. Preheat your barbecue or stovetop grill over medium/high heat.
4. Cook the fish for 5 to 7 minutes per side or until each fillet is cooked all the way through. Regularly brush the fillets with the marinade.
5. Arrange the fillets on each plate with the chives sprinkled over the top.

* Marie Callender's Famous Golden Cornbread

Makes 9 pieces

The American restaurant business has been shaped by many young entrepreneurs, so determined to realize their dreams of owning a hot dog cart or starting a restaurant that they sell everything they own to raise cash. Food lore is littered with these stories, and this one is no exception. This time the family car was sold to pay for one month's rent on a converted World War II army tent, an oven, refrigerator, rolling pin, and some hand tools. It was 1948, and that's all that Marie Callender and her family needed to make enough pies to start delivering to restaurants in Long Beach, California.

It was pies that started the company, but soon the bakeries became restaurants and they started serving meals. One of my favorites is the Famous Golden Cornbread and whipped honey butter that comes with many of the entrees. What makes this cornbread so scrumptious is its cake-like quality. The recipe here requires more flour than traditional cornbread recipes, making the finished product soft and spongy just like Marie's.

1¼ cups all-purpose flour	¾ teaspoon salt
¾ cup cornmeal	1¼ cups whole milk
2 teaspoons baking powder	¼ cup shortening
⅓ cup sugar	1 egg

Honey Butter

½ cup (1 stick) butter, softened	⅓ cup honey

1. Preheat the oven to 400 degrees F.
2. Combine the flour, cornmeal, baking powder, sugar, and salt in a medium bowl.
3. Add the milk, shortening, and egg and mix only until all the ingredients are well combined.

179

4. Pour the batter into a greased 8 × 8-inch pan.
5. Bake for 25 to 30 minutes or until the top is golden brown. Let the cornbread cool slightly before slicing it with a sharp knife into 9 pieces.
6. For the honey butter, use a mixer on high speed to whip the butter and honey together until smooth and fluffy.

✳ Marie Callender's Chicken Pot Pie

Serves 4

Menu Description: "Tender chunks of chicken with seasonings and vegetables."

All the Marie Callender's restaurants try to maintain a homestyle ambiance, kind of like being at Grandma's house for dinner. The wallcoverings reflect styles of the thirties and forties and are complemented by dark mahogany-stained, wood-paneled walls and brass fixtures. You'll also find old-fashioned furnishings, many of them throwbacks to the forties, the time of this restaurant chain's founding fifty years ago.

The menu, which features meatloaf, pot roast, and country fried steak, reflects a satisfying homestyle cuisine that today is all too rare. If you wondered whether a company that is known for its great dessert pies could make a great pot pie . . . it can.

For this recipe, try to use small 16-ounce casserole dishes that measure 4 or 5 inches across at the top. Any casserole dishes that come close to this size will probably work; the yield will vary depending on what size dishes you decide to use.

Crust

1½ cups all-purpose flour	3 tablespoons ice water
¾ teaspoon salt	⅔ cup cold butter
2 egg yolks	

Filling

1 cup sliced carrots (3 carrots)	5 tablespoons all-purpose flour
1 cup sliced celery (1 stalk)	
2 cups frozen peas	2½ cups chicken broth
1 cup chopped white onion	⅔ cup milk
4 boneless, skinless chicken breast halves	½ teaspoon salt
	Dash pepper
4 tablespoons butter	1 egg, beaten

1. Prepare the crust by sifting together the flour and salt in a medium bowl. Make a depression in the center of the flour with your hand.
2. Put the yolks and ice water into the depression. Slice the butter into tablespoon-size portions and add it into the flour depression as well.
3. Using a fork, cut the wet ingredients into the dry ingredients. When all of the flour is moistened, use your hands to finish combining the ingredients. This will ensure that the chunks of butter are well blended into the dough. Roll the dough into a ball, cover it with plastic wrap and put it into the refrigerator for 1 to 2 hours. This will make the dough easier to work with.
4. When the dough has chilled, preheat the oven to 425 degrees F and start on the filling by steaming the vegetables. Steam the carrots and celery for 5 minutes in a steamer or a saucepan with a small amount of water in the bottom. Add the frozen peas and onions and continue to steam for an additional 10 to 12 minutes or until the carrots are tender.
5. Prepare the chicken by poaching the breasts in lightly salted boiling water for 8 to 10 minutes.
6. In a separate large saucepan, melt the butter over medium heat, remove from the heat, then add the flour and whisk together until smooth. Add the chicken broth and milk and continue stirring over high heat until the mixture comes to a boil. Cook for an additional minute or so until thick, then reduce the heat to low.
7. Cut the poached chicken into large bite-size chunks and add them to the sauce. Add the salt and a dash of pepper.
8. Add the steamed vegetables to the sauce and simmer the mixture over medium/low heat for 4 to 5 minutes.
9. As the filling simmers, roll out the dough on a floured surface. Use one of the casserole dishes you plan to bake the pies in as a guide for cutting the dough. The filling will fit four 16-ounce casserole dishes perfectly, but you can use just about any size single-serving casserole dishes or oven-safe bowls for this recipe. Invert one of the dishes onto the dough and use a knife to cut around the rim. Make the cut about a half-inch larger all

of the way around to give the dough a small "lip," which you will fold over when you cover the pie. Make four of these.

10. Spoon the chicken and vegetable filling into each casserole dish and carefully cover each dish with the cut dough. Fold the edge of the dough over the edge of each dish and press firmly so that the dough sticks to the outer rim. Brush some beaten egg on the dough on each pie.

11. Bake the pies on a cookie sheet for 30 to 45 minutes or until the top crust is light brown.

✳ Marie Callender's Banana Cream Pie

Serves 6

Menu Description: "Fresh ripe bananas in our rich vanilla cream, topped with fresh whipped cream or fluffy meringue."

Bakers get to work by 5 A.M. at Marie Callender's to begin baking over 30 varieties of pies. Huge pies. Pies that weigh nearly three pounds apiece. The fresh, creamy, flaky, delicious pies that have made Marie Callender's famous in the food biz. On those mornings about 250 pies will be made at each of the 147 restaurants. Modest, I suppose, when compared with Thanksgiving Day when the stores can make up to 3,500 pies each.

For now though, we'll start with just one—banana cream pie with flaky crust, whipped cream, and slivered almonds on top. This recipe requires that you bake the crust unfilled, so you will have to use a pie weight or other oven-safe object to keep the crust from puffing up. Large pie weights are sold in many stores, or you can use small metal or ceramic weights (sold in packages) or dried beans on the crust which has first been lined with aluminum foil or parchment paper.

¼ cup butter	¼ teaspoon salt
¼ cup shortening	1 egg yolk
1¼ cups all-purpose flour	2 tablespoons ice water
1 tablespoon sugar	½ teaspoon vinegar

Filling

⅔ cup sugar	4 egg yolks, beaten
¼ cup cornstarch	1 tablespoon butter
½ teaspoon salt	2 teaspoons vanilla
2¾ cups whole milk	2 ripe bananas, sliced

Topping

1 can whipped cream	¼ cup slivered almonds

184

1. Beat together the butter and shortening until smooth and creamy and chill until firm.
2. Sift together the flour, sugar, and salt in a medium bowl.

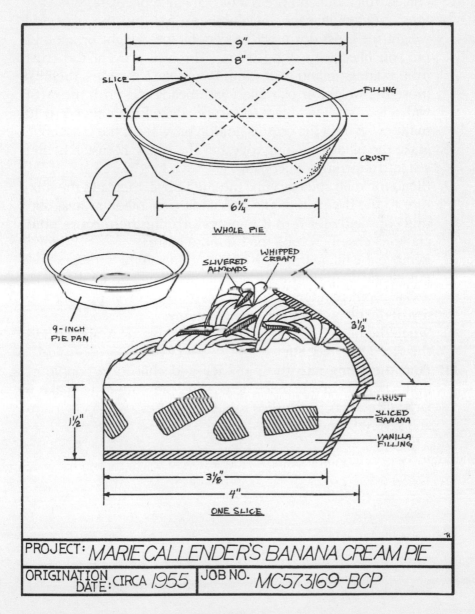

9"
8"
SLICE
FILLING
CRUST
6¼"
WHOLE PIE

9-INCH PIE PAN

SLIVERED ALMONDS
WHIPPED CREAM
3½"
CRUST
SLICED BANANA
VANILLA FILLING
1½"
3⅛"
4"
ONE SLICE

PROJECT: *MARIE CALLENDER'S BANANA CREAM PIE*
ORIGINATION DATE: CIRCA *1955*   JOB NO. *MC573169-BCP*

3. Using a fork, cut the butter and shortening into the dry ingredients, until the mixture has a consistent texture. Mix egg yolk, ice water, and vinegar into the dough, then form it into a ball and refrigerate it for 1 hour so that it will be easier to work with.
4. Preheat the oven to 450 degrees F. When the dough has chilled, roll it out and press it into a 9-inch pie plate.
5. Press parchment paper or aluminum foil into the crust and weight the crust down with a ceramic pie weight or another pie pan filled with dried beans. This will prevent the crust from puffing up and distorting. Bake for 15 minutes, then remove the weight or pan filled with beans and prick the crust with a fork to allow steam to escape. Bake for another 5 to 10 minutes, or until the crust is golden brown. Let the crust cool.
6. Make the filling by sifting together the sugar, cornstarch, and salt into a medium saucepan.
7. Blend the milk and eggs in a medium bowl, then add the mixture to the dry ingredients and cook over medium heat stirring constantly for 6 to 8 minutes or until the mixture boils and thickens, then cook for 1 minute more.
8. Remove the filling from the heat, and mix in the vanilla.
9. Put plastic wrap on the surface of the filling and let it cool to about room temperature. The plastic wrap will prevent the top of the filling from becoming gummy.
10. When the filling has cooled, remove the plastic wrap and add the sliced bananas. Stir.
11. Pour the filling into the pie shell and chill for a couple of hours before serving. Slice across the pie 3 times to make 6 large slices. Serve each slice topped with fresh whipped cream and slivered almonds.

✳ Olive Garden Italian Salad Dressing

Makes 1½ cups

In the 1970s, food conglomerate General Mills set out to expand its growing restaurant business. A research team was organized to study the market, and to conduct interviews with potential customers on what they would want in a restaurant. Seven years later, in 1982, the first Olive Garden restaurant opened its doors in Orlando, Florida. Today it is the number one Italian restaurant chain in the country with over 470 stores.

One of the favorites at the Olive Garden is an item that isn't even mentioned in the menu: the Italian salad dressing served on the house salad that comes with every meal. The dressing became so popular that the chain now sells it by the bottle "to go" in each restaurant. Now you can make a version of the dressing for yourself that tastes just like the original, but will cost much less. The secret to thickening this dressing is to use dry pectin, a natural ingredient often used to thicken jams and jellies. Pectin can be found in most stores in the aisle with baking and cooking supplies or near the canning items.

½ cup white vinegar
⅓ cup water
⅓ cup vegetable oil
¼ cup corn syrup
2½ tablespoons grated
    Romano cheese
2 tablespoons dry pectin
2 tablespoons beaten egg
    or egg substitute

1¼ teaspoons salt
1 teaspoon lemon juice
½ teaspoon minced garlic
¼ teaspoon dried parsley
    flakes
Pinch of dried oregano
Pinch of crushed red
    pepper flakes

Combine all of the ingredients with a mixer on medium speed or in a blender on low speed for 30 seconds. Chill at least 1 hour. Serve over mixed greens or use as a marinade.

✳ Olive Garden
Hot Artichoke-Spinach Dip

Serves 4 as an appetizer

Menu Description: *"A creamy hot dip of artichokes, spinach and parmesan with pasta chips."*

It's interesting to note that just about every aspect of the Olive Garden restaurants was developed from consumer research conducted in a corporate think tank by the General Mills corporation. Restaurant-goers were questioned about preferences such as the type of food to be served, the appearance and atmosphere of the restaurant, even the color of the candle holders on each table. The large tables and the comfy chairs on rollers that you see today at the Olive Garden restaurants came out of these vigorous research sessions.

I'm not sure if this dish came from those sessions, but according to servers at the Olive Garden, the Hot Artichoke-Spinach Dip is one of the most requested appetizers on the menu. The restaurant serves the dip with chips made from fried pasta, but you can serve this version of the popular appetizer with just about any type of crackers, chips, or toasted Italian bread, like bruschetta.

1 cup chopped artichoke hearts (canned or frozen and thawed)	½ cup grated Parmesan cheese
	½ teaspoon crushed red pepper flakes
½ cup frozen chopped spinach, thawed	¼ teaspoon salt
8 ounces cream cheese	⅛ teaspoon garlic powder
	Dash ground pepper

On the Side

Crackers	Sliced, toasted bread
Chips	

1. Boil the spinach and artichoke hearts in a cup of water in a small saucepan over medium heat until tender, about 10 minutes. Drain in a colander when done.

2. Heat the cream cheese in a small bowl in the microwave set on high for 1 minute. Or, use a saucepan to heat the cheese over medium heat just until hot.
3. Add the spinach and artichoke hearts to the cream cheese and stir well.
4. Add the remaining ingredients to the cream cheese and combine. Serve hot with crackers, chips, or toasted bread for dipping.

Tidbits

It's easy to make a lighter version of this dip by using a reduced fat cream cheese in the same measurement.

✳ Olive Garden Toscana Soup

Serves 4 as an appetizer, 2 as an entree

Menu Description: "Spicy sausage, russet potatoes, and cavolo greens in a light creamy broth."

For two years after the first Olive Garden restaurant opened in 1982, operators were still tweaking the restaurant's physical appearance and the food that was served. Even the tomato sauce was changed as many as 25 times.

This soup blends the flavors of potatoes, kale, and Italian sausage in a slightly spicy chicken and cream broth. When I first tried the soup at the restaurant I was surprised at how good it was. I'd never had any soup with the leafy, healthy, spinach-like kale in it (found in most produce sections), and the combination of flavors was addicting. When you try this version for yourself I think you'll agree.

2¾ cups chicken stock or broth	½ pound spicy Italian sausage
¼ cup heavy cream	¼ teaspoon salt
1 medium russet potato	¼ teaspoon crushed red pepper flakes
2 cups chopped kale	

1. Combine the stock and cream in a saucepan over medium heat.
2. Slice the unpeeled potato into ¼-inch slices, then quarter the slices and add them to the soup.
3. Add the kale.
4. Grill or sauté the sausage. When cooked and cooled, cut the sausage at an angle into slices about ½ inch thick. Add the sausage to the soup.
5. Add the spices and let the soup simmer for about 2 hours. Stir occasionally.

✳ Olive Garden Alfredo Pasta

Serves 2 to 3 as an entree

Menu Description: *"Our classically rich blend of cream, butter and parmesan cheese with a hint of garlic."*

The Alfredo Pasta served at the Olive Garden is a tasty, classic recipe. Although rich and creamy, the simplicity of this recipe made it hard for me to resist. This is one of those fail-safe recipes that can be made quickly and easily with just a few ingredients.

Serve this dish with a Toscana soup appetizer and some garlic bread and you've got a tasty meal just like one you might get at the restaurant chain—except this version will cost less, you can enjoy it in the comfort of home, and you won't have to tip.

½ cup (1 stick) butter
2 cups heavy cream
⅛ teaspoon garlic powder
⅛ teaspoon ground black pepper

1 12-ounce box fettuccine pasta (or your choice of pasta)
¼ cup grated Parmesan cheese

1. Melt the butter in a medium saucepan over medium heat.
2. Add the cream, garlic powder, and pepper and simmer for 10 to 12 minutes or until thick.
3. At the same time, bring 4 to 6 quarts of water to a boil and add the pasta.
4. When the Alfredo sauce has reached your desired consistency, stir in the Parmesan cheese.
5. When the pasta is cooked, drain it. Serve the pasta on plates with Alfredo sauce poured over the top.

✳ Outback Steakhouse Bloomin' Onion

Serves 2 to 4 as an appetizer or snack

Menu Description: *"An Outback Ab-original from Russell's Marina Bay."*

If you go to an Outback Steakhouse expecting exotic Aussie prairie food that someone like Crocodile Dundee would have enjoyed, you're gonna be a bit disappointed, mate. Except for a little Australia-themed paraphernalia on the walls, like boomerangs and pictures of kangaroos, the restaurant chain is about as "down under" as McDonald's is Irish. The three founders, Tim Gannon, Chris Sullivan, and Bob Basham, are all U.S. boys. And the menu, which is about 60 percent beef, contains mainly American fare with cute Australian names like The Melbourne, Jackeroo Chops, and Chicken on the Barbie.

The founders say they chose the Aussie theme because "Most Australians are fun-loving and gregarious people and very casual people. We thought that's exactly the kind of friendliness and atmosphere we want to have in our restaurants."

In only six years, Outback Steakhouse has become our number one steakhouse chain—in part because of the Bloomin' Onion: a large, deep-fried onion sliced to look like a flower in bloom that was created by one of the restaurant's founders. What makes this appetizer so appealing besides its flowery appearance is the onion's crispy spiced coating, along with the delicious dipping sauce, cleverly presented in the center of the onion.

Although the restaurant uses a special device to make the slicing process easier, you can make the incisions with a sharp knife. It just takes a steady hand and a bit of care.

Dipping Sauce

½ cup mayonnaise
2 teaspoons ketchup
2 tablespoons cream-style horseradish
¼ teaspoon paprika

¼ teaspoon salt
⅛ teaspoon dried oregano
Dash ground black pepper
Dash cayenne pepper

192

The Onion

1 egg	1/4 teaspoon dried oregano
1 cup milk	1/8 teaspoon dried thyme
1 cup all-purpose flour	1/8 teaspoon cumin
1 1/2 teaspoons salt	1 jumbo sweet yellow or
1 1/2 teaspoons cayenne pepper	white onion (3/4 pound
1 teaspoon paprika	or more)
1/2 teaspoon ground black	Vegetable oil for frying
pepper	

1. Prepare the dipping sauce by combining all of the ingredients in a small bowl. Keep the sauce covered in your refrigerator until needed.
2. Beat the egg and combine it with the milk in a medium bowl big enough to hold the onion.
3. In a separate bowl, combine the flour, salt, peppers, paprika, oregano, thyme, and cumin.
4. Now it's time to slice the onion—this is the trickiest step. First slice 3/4 inch to 1 inch off the top and bottom of the onion. Remove the papery skin. Use a thin knife to cut a 1-inch diameter core out of the middle of the onion. Now use a very sharp, large knife to slice the onion several times down the center to create the "petals" of the completed onion. First slice through the center of the onion to about three-fourths of the way down. Turn the onion 90 degrees and slice it again in an "x" across the first slice. Keep slicing the sections in half, very carefully, until you've cut the onion 16 times. Do not cut down to the bottom. The last 8 slices are a little hairy, just use a steady hand and don't worry if your onion doesn't look like a perfect flower. It'll still taste good.
5. Spread the "petals" of the onion apart. The onion sections tend to stick together, so you'll want to separate them to make coating easier. To help separate the "petals," plunge the onion into boiling water for 1 minute, and then into cold water.
6. Dip the onion in the milk mixture, and then coat it liberally with the dry ingredients. Again separate the "petals" and sprinkle the dry coating between them. Once you're sure the onion is well-coated, dip it back into the wet mixture and into the dry coating again. This double dipping makes sure you have a well-coated onion because some of the coating tends to wash off

193

when you fry. Let the onion rest in the refrigerator for at least 15 minutes while you get the oil ready.

7. Heat oil in a deep fryer or deep pot to 350 degrees F. Make sure you use enough oil to completely cover the onion when it fries.

8. Fry the onion right side up in the oil for 10 minutes or until it turns brown.

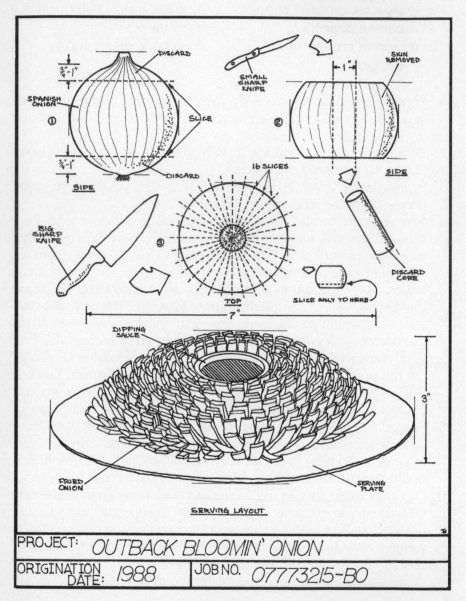

SERVING LAYOUT

PROJECT: *OUTBACK BLOOMIN' ONION*

ORIGINATION DATE: *1988*   JOB NO. *07773215-BO*

9. When the onion has browned, remove it from the oil and let it drain on a rack or paper towels.
10. Open the onion wider from the center so that you can put a small dish of the dipping sauce in the center. You may also use plain ketchup.

✳ Outback Steakhouse
Gold Coast Coconut Shrimp

Serves 4 as an appetizer

Menu Description: "Six colossal shrimp dipped in beer batter,
rolled in coconut, deep-fried to a golden brown and
served with marmalade sauce."

The three founders of Outback Steakhouse are an experienced
lot of restaurateurs. Tim Gannon, Chris Sullivan, and Bob Basham
had each worked for the Steak & Ale chain of restaurants at one
time or another, as well as other large casual dining chains. When
the three got together and decided they wanted to open a few
restaurants in the Tampa, Florida, area, they had modest ambitions.

Basham told *Food & Beverage* magazine, "We figured if we divided up the profits with what we thought we could make out of
five or six restaurants, we could have a very nice lifestyle and play a
lot of golf." The first six restaurants opened within 13 months.
Eight years later the chain had grown to over 300 restaurants, and
the three men now have a very, very nice lifestyle indeed.

Coconut Shrimp is a sweet and crispy fried appetizer not found
on most other menus, especially with the delicious marmalade
sauce. Outback servers claim it's a top seller.

At the restaurant chain, you get six of these shrimp to serve two
as an appetizer, but since we're taking the time to make the batter
and use all of that oil, I thought I'd up the yield to a dozen shrimp
to serve four as an appetizer. If you don't want to make that many,
you can use the same recipe with fewer shrimp and save the leftover batter to make more later or just toss it out.

1 **cup flat beer**	2 **tablespoons sugar**
1 **cup self-rising flour**	½ **teaspoon salt**
2 **cups sweetened coconut flakes (1 7-ounce package)**	12 **jumbo shrimp**
	Vegetable oil for frying
	Paprika

196

Marmalade Sauce (for Dipping)

½ cup orange marmalade
2 teaspoons stone-ground
    mustard (with whole-
    grain mustard seed)

1 teaspoon prepared
   horseradish
Dash salt

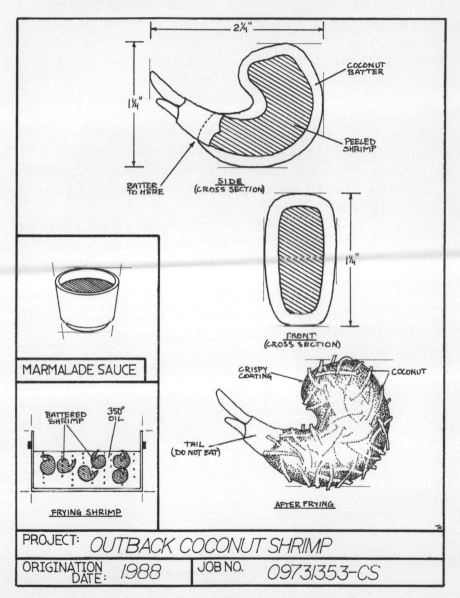

2¼"

1¼"

COCONUT
BATTER

PEELED
SHRIMP

BATTER
TO HERE

SIDE
(CROSS SECTION)

1¾"

FRONT
(CROSS SECTION)

MARMALADE SAUCE

BATTERED
SHRIMP

350°
OIL

FRYING SHRIMP

CRISPY
COATING

COCONUT

TAIL
(DO NOT EAT)

AFTER FRYING

PROJECT: OUTBACK COCONUT SHRIMP

ORIGINATION
DATE: 1988

JOB NO. 09731353-CS

1. For the batter, use an electric mixer to combine the beer, flour, ½ cup coconut flakes, sugar, and salt in a medium-size bowl. Mix well, then cover and refrigerate at least 1 hour.
2. Prepare your marmalade sauce by combining all four ingredients in a small bowl. Cover and refrigerate this for at least 1 hour as well.
3. Prepare the shrimp by deveining and peeling off the shell back to the tail. Leave the last segment of the shell plus the tailfins as a handle.
4. When the batter is ready, preheat oil in a deep pot or deep fryer to about 350 degrees F. Use enough oil to completely cover the shrimp. Pour the remainder of the coconut into a shallow bowl.
5. Be sure the shrimp are dry before battering. Sprinkle each shrimp lightly with paprika before the next step.
6. Dip one shrimp at a time into the batter, coating generously. Drop the battered shrimp into the coconut and roll it around so that it is well coated.
7. Fry four shrimp at a time for 2 to 3 minutes or until the shrimp become golden brown. You may have to flip the shrimp over halfway through cooking time. Drain on paper towels briefly before serving with marmalade sauce on the side.

✳ Outback Steakhouse Walkabout Soup

Serves 4 as an appetizer

Menu Description: "A unique presentation of an Australian favorite. Reckon!"

Here's a great way to start off dinner. The menu claims the Walkabout Soup is an Australian favorite. While that may or may not be true, this creamy onion soup with two types of cheese on top is at least a favorite of mine. If you can boil water and slice onions, you'll have no problem with this easy-to-make version of the chain's top secret formula.

8 cups water	1 cup heavy cream
8 beef bouillon cubes	1¼ cups shredded Cheddar
3 medium white onions	cheese
1 teaspoon salt	¼ cup shredded Monterey
1 teaspoon black pepper	Jack cheese
¾ cup all-purpose flour	

1. Heat the water to boiling in a large pan. Add the bouillon cubes and dissolve.
2. Cut the onions into thin slices, then quarter the slices. Add to the broth.
3. Add salt and pepper.
4. Bring the mixture back to boiling, then turn the heat down and simmer, uncovered, for 1 hour.
5. While stirring, sift the flour into the soup. Continue to stir if any large lumps of flour develop. Be careful when you stir; aggressive agitation or using a whisk may tear the onions apart. As the soup continues to cook, any lumps should dissolve.
6. After 30 minutes of additional simmering, add the cream and 1 cup Cheddar cheese. Continue to simmer the soup for another 5 to 10 minutes.
7. Serve the soup hot after sprinkling a tablespoon each of shredded Monterey Jack and Cheddar on top.

199

✳ Outback Steakhouse Alice Springs Chicken

Serves 4 as an entree

Menu Description: "Grilled chicken breast and bacon
smothered in mushrooms, melted Monterey Jack and Cheddar cheeses,
with honey mustard sauce."

In the late eighties, as the public's concern about eating beef
was growing, the restaurant industry saw a big shift toward chicken
meals. In the midst of a poultry-crazy country, that last thing you'd
expect anyone to do is open a steakhouse. But that's exactly what
the boys who founded Outback Steakhouse did. And by the time
their restaurant had become the sixth largest dinnerhouse chain
in the country, they had proven that what many people still want
is a big honkin' slab of beef.

With a menu dominated by beef items, it's nice to find that the
restaurant can do great things with chicken meals as well, such as
the Alice Springs Chicken. You'll love the mushrooms, bacon,
cheese, and honey mustard piled on a chicken breast that's been
grilled on the "barbie."

Honey Mustard Marinade

½ cup Grey Poupon Dijon
    mustard
½ cup honey

1½ teaspoons vegetable oil
½ teaspoon lemon juice

4 skinless, boneless chicken
   breast halves
1 tablespoon vegetable oil
2 cups sliced mushrooms
   (10 to 12 mushrooms)
2 tablespoons butter
Salt
Pepper

Paprika
8 slices bacon, cooked
1 cup shredded Monterey
   Jack cheese
1 cup shredded Cheddar
   cheese
2 teaspoons finely chopped
   fresh parsley

1. Use an electric mixer to combine the Dijon mustard, honey, 1½ teaspoons oil, and lemon juice in a small bowl. Whip the mixture for about 30 seconds.
2. Pour about two-thirds of the marinade over the chicken breasts and marinate them, covered, in the refrigerator for about 2 hours. Chill the remaining marinade until later.

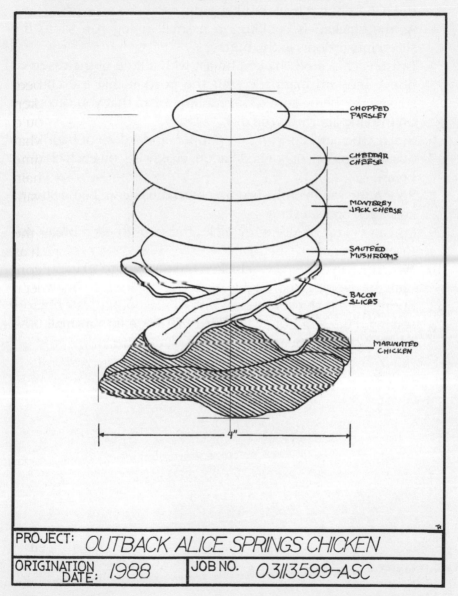

CHOPPED PARSLEY

CHEDDAR CHEESE

MONTEREY JACK CHEESE

SAUTÉED MUSHROOMS

BACON SLICES

MARINATED CHICKEN

4"

PROJECT: *OUTBACK ALICE SPRINGS CHICKEN*

ORIGINATION DATE: *1988*   JOB NO. *03113599-ASC*

3. After the chicken has marinated, preheat the oven to 375 degrees F and heat up an ovenproof frying pan large enough to hold all four breasts and 1 tablespoon of oil over medium heat. (If you don't have an ovenproof skillet, transfer the chicken to a baking dish for baking.) Sear the chicken in the pan for 3 to 4 minutes per side or until golden brown. Remove the pan from the heat, but keep the chicken in the pan.
4. As the chicken is cooking, in a small frying pan sauté the sliced mushrooms in the butter.
5. Brush each seared chicken breast with a little of the reserved honey mustard marinade (*not* the portion that the chicken soaked in), being sure to save a little extra that you can serve on the side later with the dish.
6. Season the chicken with salt, pepper, and a dash of paprika.
7. Stack two pieces of cooked bacon, crosswise, on each chicken breast.
8. Spoon the sautéed mushrooms onto the bacon, being sure to coat each breast evenly.
9. Spread ¼ cup of Monterey Jack cheese onto each breast followed by ¼ cup of Cheddar.
10. Bake the pan of prepared chicken breasts for 7 to 10 minutes or until the cheese is thoroughly melted and starting to bubble.
11. Sprinkle each chicken breast with ½ teaspoon parsley before serving. Put extra honey mustard marinade into a small bowl to serve on the side.

✳ Perkins Family Restaurants Potato Pancakes

Serves 3 to 4 as a breakfast or side dish

Menu Description: "Hearty pancakes made with grated potatoes, onions and parsley."

When Matt and Ivan Perkins tasted the food at Smitty's Pancake House in Seattle, they were smitten. Soon they had purchased the rights to William Smith's recipes, which had been perfected at his renowned restaurant since it opened just after World War II. In 1958, the brothers realized their dream and opened a Smitty's restaurant of their own in Cincinnati, Ohio. When the brothers decided to give the chain an identity all its own, all of the Smitty's were changed to Perkins, and business continued to thrive through the years.

If you've never tried potato pancakes from Perkins or any restaurant, now's the time. This is a tasty classic, breakfast recipe that doesn't necessarily have to be for breakfast. I've given you the option to make the pancakes with frozen hash brown potatoes or with fresh potatoes you shred by hand. The fresh potatoes obviously taste better, but if you're in a rush, go with frozen. It may sound strange if you haven't tried it, but maple or maple-flavored syrup goes great on these hotcakes. At least I think so. You may just want some butter and powdered sugar on top.

1 cup all-purpose flour
1 cup whole milk
4 eggs
3 tablespoons butter, melted
3 tablespoons sugar
¼ teaspoon baking powder
½ teaspoon salt

1 tablespoon chopped fresh parsley
1 tablespoon minced onion
2½ cups frozen hash browns (defrosted) or shredded fresh potatoes (3 to 4)

On the Side

Butter   Syrup

1. Combine all of the ingredients, except the potatoes, in a large mixing bowl. Beat by hand or with an electric mixer until smooth.
2. Add the potatoes to the batter and mix by hand until the potatoes are well combined.
3. Let the batter rest while you preheat a skillet or griddle to about medium heat. Grease the pan with a little butter. You may also use nonstick spray.
4. Ladle ¼-cup dollops of batter into the pan. Cook as many at a time as will fit comfortably in your pan. Cook each pancake for 1½ to 2 minutes per side until brown. Serve in a fanned-out stack with a pat of butter on top. Serve syrup on the side, if desired.

Tidbits

Because fresh shredded potatoes have more moisture than frozen, you may need to add a couple tablespoons more flour to the batter if you decide to shred your own spuds.

✳ Perkins Family Restaurants Granny's Country Omelette

Serves 2

Menu Description: "Brimming with a blend of diced ham, onions, crisp celery and green peppers folded into a rich, luscious cheese sauce. With hashed browns tucked inside."

The same year that Matt and Ivan Perkins opened their first diner, they started selling franchise rights to other entrepreneurs. Back then, the name for the chain west of the Mississippi was still Smitty's, and to the east it became Perkins Pancake House. Soon, the name was changed to Perkins Cake & Steak. But that wouldn't last either. In the seventies the western chain of Smitty's and the eastern Perkins consolidated, and Perkins Family Restaurants, as we know it today, was born.

Secret breakfast recipes are what originally made Perkins famous. The trademarked Granny's Country Omelette is a popular menu selection from the "Premium Omelettes" column. It's a clever design for an omelette with the hash browns hidden away inside the folded eggs in a compartment separate from the other filling ingredients. The trick here is getting the folding right. I've tried to describe it as clearly as possible in the preparation steps, but if that confuses you, consult the illustration—as they say, "a picture is worth a thousand words."

1 cup frozen hash browns, uncooked

2 tablespoons butter

½ green bell pepper, diced (½ cup)

½ red bell pepper, diced (½ cup)

2 slices white onion, diced (½ cup)

2 tablespoons minced celery

5 ounces ham, diced (½ cup)

½ pound Velveeta cheese spread

3 tablespoons milk

6 large eggs

Salt

1. Cook the hash browns following the directions on the package.
2. Sauté the vegetables in 1 tablespoon of butter over medium/high heat. Cut the ham into very small cubes and toss it in with the vegetables. After 3 to 5 minutes, when the ham starts to brown, it's ready.

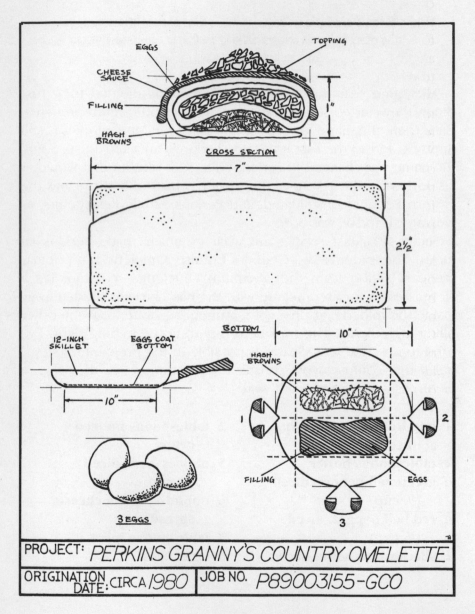

3. Prepare the cheese sauce while the ham and vegetables are cooking. In a small saucepan, combine the cheese spread with the milk over low heat. Stir occasionally until melted. Be careful not to burn it.

4. Use a 12-inch frying pan or omelette pan for making the omelette. While the pan is preheating over medium heat, beat the eggs in a mixing bowl until smooth and creamy, but not foamy. Put ½ tablespoon of butter into the middle of the pan and swirl it around. Pour half of the beaten eggs into the buttered pan and swirl the pan around to coat the entire bottom with eggs. You want only a thin layer of eggs in the pan. This may require that you use a bit less than half of the eggs, so you may have some beaten egg left over in the end. Salt the eggs.

5. When the eggs have cooked for a minute or so, pour a quarter of the sautéed filling onto the eggs in a vertical line to the left of the middle, leaving enough room so that you will be able to fold over the top and bottom. Spoon half of the hash browns parallel to the filling just to the right of the middle. Fold the top and bottom of the omelette in, then fold the omelette from the left, over the top of the vegetable and ham filling. Fold the omelette once again, this time from the right, over the hash browns, then fold it one more time in the same direction, into a neat little package. Let it cook for another minute or so.

6. Carefully slide the omelette out of the pan, seam-side down, onto a plate. Put this omelette into a 250 degrees F oven to keep warm until the second omelette is done. Cook the other omelette.

7. When both omelettes are done, pour a generous helping of cheese sauce over each one and sprinkle the remaining veggies and ham over the cheese sauce.

✳ Perkins Family Restaurants Country Club Omelette

Serves 2

Menu Description: "Oven-roasted turkey breast, real bacon pieces, green onions and fresh tomatoes. In a delicate hollandaise sauce."

This restaurant chain gained a large following early on for its homestyle breakfast menu. Today, even though you can eat from the breakfast menu whenever you like, customers are picking from the lunch and dinner selections just about as often.

Since it was originally the breakfast selection that made this chain famous, I'm offering another great omelette recipe. The Country Club Omelette answers the question "What do you get when you cross a club sandwich with three eggs?" Now you can have your own version of this delicious omelette for breakfast, lunch, or dinner.

Hollandaise Sauce

½ cup butter, softened
3 egg yolks
1 tablespoon lemon juice
½ teaspoon sugar
⅛ teaspoon onion powder

⅛ teaspoon salt
Dash paprika
Dash white pepper
½ cup boiling water

8 ounces deli-sliced roasted turkey breast
4 slices bacon, cooked
1 tomato
6 large eggs

1 tablespoon butter
Salt
2 tablespoons chopped green onion

1. For the hollandaise sauce, you'll need a double boiler. Cream the butter in a small bowl, then add the egg yolks one at a time and beat with an electric mixer. Add the remaining ingredients, except for the boiling water, and mix. Add the boiling water, slowly, a little bit at a time, and stir until creamy; then

pour the sauce into the top of a double boiler over boiling water. Stir continuously until thick, then turn off the heat and let the sauce keep warm over the hot water until the omelettes are done.

2. Cut the turkey breast into nickel-size pieces, crumble the bacon, and dice the tomato. Combine the three ingredients in a

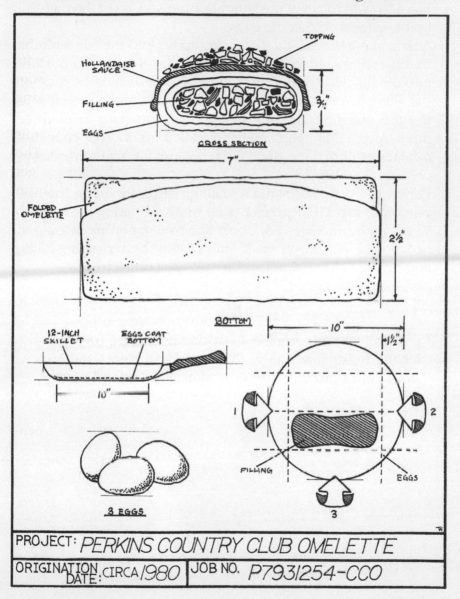

PROJECT: *PERKINS COUNTRY CLUB OMELETTE*

ORIGINATION DATE: CIRCA *1980* JOB NO. *P7931254-CCO*

small skillet over low heat. You just want these ingredients to heat up while the eggs are being prepared.

3. Crack the eggs into a mixing bowl and beat by hand or with an electric mixer until smooth and creamy, but not foamy.

4. Heat a 12-inch skillet over medium heat. Add ½ tablespoon butter to the pan and swirl it around. Pour half of the eggs into the pan and swirl to cover the entire bottom surface of the pan and up the edge a bit. Salt the eggs.

5. After a minute or so add the green onions into the pan with the bacon, turkey, and tomato. Then pour one-third of the mixture into the omelette, just to the left or right of the center. Arrange the filling in a vertical line, leaving room so that you can fold in the top and bottom, and then roll the omelette over three times. After folding the omelette, cook it for another couple of minutes or until done. Slide the omelette out, seam side down, on a serving plate.

6. Repeat the process for the remaining omelette. Keep the first one warm in a 250 degrees F oven while preparing the second.

7. When both omelettes are done, spoon a generous helping of hollandaise sauce over each one. Divide the remaining filling and spoon it over the hollandaise on each omelette.

Tidbits

If you like, you can simplify the recipe by using a packaged dry mix for the hollandaise sauce. I've found that Knorr and McCormick make great products that taste similar to Perkins' sauce.

✳ Pizza Hut
Original Stuffed Crust Pizza

Serves 3 to 4

Menu Description: "This unique thinner crust has a ring of cheese baked into the edge so you get cheese in the very last bite of every slice."

Brothers Dan and Frank Carney have dear old Mom to thank for helping them to become founders of the world's largest pizza chain. It was in 1958 that a family friend approached the two brothers with the idea of opening a pizza parlor, and it was the brothers' mother who lent them the $600 it took to purchase some second-hand equipment and to rent a small building. There, in the Carneys' hometown of Wichita, Kansas, the first Pizza Hut opened its doors. By 1966, there were 145 Pizza Hut restaurants doing a booming business around the country with the help of the promotional musical jingle "Putt-Putt to Pizza Hut." Today the chain is made up of more than 10,000 restaurants, delivery–carry out units, and kiosks in all 50 states and 82 foreign countries.

Introduced in 1995, the Stuffed Crust Pizza, which includes sticks of mozzarella string cheese loaded into the crust before cooking, increased business at Pizza Hut by 37 percent. Because the outer crust is filled with cheese, the chain designed a special dough formula that does not rise as high as the original. It's best to prepare your Top Secret Recipe version of this delicious crust a day before you plan to cook the pizza so that the dough can rest while the gluten in the flour forms a texture just like the original.

Crust

¾ cup warm water (105 degrees to 115 degrees F)	1 tablespoon sugar
	2¼ cups bread flour
	1½ teaspoons salt
1¼ teaspoons yeast	1½ tablespoons olive oil

211

Sauce

1 15-ounce can tomato sauce
¼ teaspoon dried oregano
¼ teaspoon dried basil leaves
¼ teaspoon dried thyme
¼ teaspoon garlic powder
¼ teaspoon salt

⅛ teaspoon ground black pepper
1 bay leaf
Dash onion powder
½ teaspoon lemon juice

8 1-ounce mozzarella string cheese sticks

1½ cups shredded mozzarella

Toppings (your choice of . . .)

pepperoni slices, chopped onions, sliced mushrooms, sliced black olives, sliced jalapeños (nacho slices), sliced green peppers, pineapple chunks, Italian sausage, sliced tomatoes, sliced ham, anchovies

1. First prepare the dough for the crust. I suggest you prepare the crust one day prior to baking the pizza. To get the best dough you need to allow it to rise in your refrigerator overnight. This procedure will produce a great commercial-style crust.

   Combine the warm water, sugar, and yeast in a small bowl or measuring cup and stir until the yeast and sugar have dissolved. Let the mixture sit for about 5 minutes. Foam should begin building up on the surface. If it doesn't, either the water was too hot or the yeast was dead. Throw it out and start again.

2. In a large bowl, sift together the flour and salt. Make a depression in the center of the flour and pour in the yeast mixture. Add the oil.

3. Use a fork to stir the liquid in the center of the flour. Slowly draw in more flour, a little bit at a time, until you have to use your hands to completely combine all of the ingredients into a ball.

4. Dust a clean, flat surface with flour, and with the heel of your hands, knead the dough on this surface until it seems to have a smooth, consistent texture. This should take around 10 minutes. Rub a light coating of oil on the dough, then put it into a tightly covered container and in a warm place to rise for 2 hours or until it

212

has doubled in size. When it has doubled in size, punch the dough down, put it back into the covered container and into the refrigerator overnight. If you don't have time for that, you can use the crust at this point. But without the long rest it just won't have the same texture as the original.

5. You can prepare the pizza sauce ahead of time as well, storing it in the refrigerator until you are ready to make the pizza. Simply combine the tomato sauce with the spices and lemon juice in a small saucepan over medium heat. Heat the sauce until it starts to bubble, then turn the heat down and simmer, covered, for 30 to 60 minutes until it reaches the thickness you like. When the sauce has cooled, store it in the refrigerator in a tightly sealed container.

6. About an hour or so before you are ready to make your pizza, take the dough out of the refrigerator so that it will warm up to room temperature.

Preheat the oven to 475 degrees F.

Roll the dough out on a floured surface until it is 18 inches across. Put the dough on a pizza pan that has either been greased or has a sprinkling of cornmeal on it. This will prevent your pizza from sticking. Score the pizza dough several times with a fork so that it doesn't bubble up when baked.

7. Place a ring of the string cheese sticks, end to end, around the edge of the dough, an inch in from the edge.

8. Use water on your fingertips or on a brush to moisten the outer edge of the dough, all of the way around so that it will stick when folded over. Fold the dough up and over the cheese and press it down onto itself, sealing it tightly. Form a nice, round crust as you seal the cheese inside. Lightly brush the top of the folded dough with olive oil all of the way around the edge.

9. Now spread about a cup of the pizza sauce on the crust (you will likely have enough sauce left over for another pie later). As you spread the sauce onto the crust, be sure to spread sauce all of the way to the folded edge, enough to hide that seam you made when folding the crust over the cheese.

10. Spread the toppings other than pepperoni, sausage, ham, and olives on the pizza sauce. Sprinkle the shredded mozzarella

213

onto the sauce and any olives or meat toppings you wish on top of the cheese.

11. Bake the pizza for 12 to 16 minutes or until the crust begins to turn dark brown and the cheese develops dark spots.

12. Slice the pizza 4 times through the center, making 8 slices.

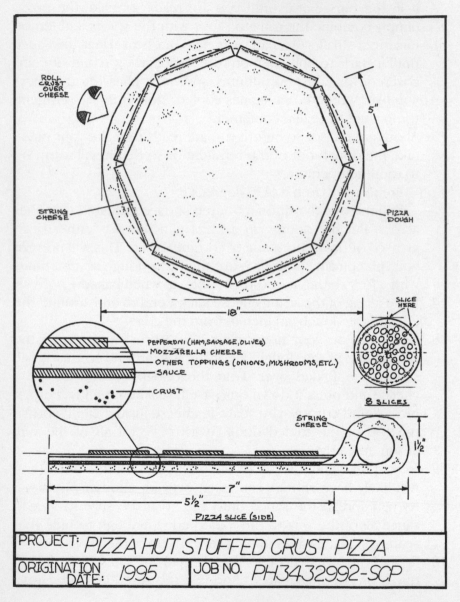

ROLL CRUST OVER CHEESE

5"

STRING CHEESE

PIZZA DOUGH

18"

PEPPERONI (HAM, SAUSAGE, OLIVES)
MOZZARELLA CHEESE
OTHER TOPPINGS (ONIONS, MUSHROOMS, ETC.)
SAUCE
CRUST

SLICE HERE

8 SLICES

STRING CHEESE

1½"

7"

5½"

PIZZA SLICE (SIDE)

PROJECT: PIZZA HUT STUFFED CRUST PIZZA

ORIGINATION DATE: 1995   JOB NO. PH3432992-SCP

✳ Pepperoni & Cheese
Stuffed Crust Pizza

Serves 3 to 4

After the sales success of the Original Stuffed Crust Pizza, Pizza Hut developed a variation which includes slices of pepperoni along with the gooey cheese in the crust of each pizza slice. The technique is very simple. Just place a slice of pepperoni every inch or so around the edge onto the dough where you will place the string cheese sticks. Each string cheese stick should be placed on top of the pepperoni slices and then the dough is folded over the cheese the same way as in the original recipe. The pepperoni slices will curl over the cheese sticks as you fold the dough over. Top and bake your pizza as described in the previous recipe. *Voilà!*

Tidbits

The kneading process is easy with a bread machine if you have one. Prepare the yeast, water, and sugar mixture, then add the flour, salt, and oil to the bread machine baking pan. When the yeast mixture becomes foamy on top, pour it into the baking pan and put the machine on the "dough" setting. When the dough is done, seal it up in a container and place it in the fridge overnight.

✳ Pizza Hut
TripleDecker Pizza

Serves 3 to 4

Menu Description: "We start with a thin layer of crust, then we lay down a luscious layer of our six-cheese blend and seal it in with another thin layer of crust. We pile on your favorite Pizza Hut toppings, more cheese and bake it to gooey perfection."

You might be as surprised as I was to learn that Pizza Hut uses 2.5 percent of all the milk produced in the U.S. every year for the cheese used on the pizzas. We're talking about a lot of pizzas here—1.3 million served every day. The cheese production alone requires a herd of 250,000 dairy cows producing at full capacity 365 days a year!

Certainly even more overworked cows had to be recruited to produce the additional cheese needed for this gooey new creation. This special pizza is made with two crispy cracker-like crusts that have a hidden layer of six cheeses cooked between them. Because this pizza requires two crusts, Pizza Hut created a dough that does not rise as much as the dough used in their other pizzas. This version has been adapted from a classic recipe for soda crackers. The finished product is surely the perfect pizza for people who think they just don't get enough cheese in their diet.

Crust

- ¾ teaspoon yeast
- 1 cup warm water (105 degrees to 115 degrees F)
- 3¾ cups all-purpose flour
- 2 teaspoons salt
- ½ teaspoon baking soda
- 3 tablespoons shortening
- ¼ cup milk

Sauce

- 1 15-ounce can tomato sauce
- ¼ teaspoon dried oregano
- ¼ teaspoon dried basil leaves
- ¼ teaspoon dried thyme
- ¼ teaspoon garlic powder
- ¼ teaspoon salt
- ⅛ teaspoon ground black pepper
- 1 bay leaf
- ½ teaspoon lemon juice
- Dash onion powder

216

Six-Cheese Blend

⅓ cup shredded Cheddar cheese

⅓ cup shredded Monterey Jack cheese

½ cup shredded mozzarella cheese

2 tablespoons shredded provolone

1 tablespoon grated Parmesan cheese

1 tablespoon grated Romano cheese

1½ cups shredded mozzarella cheese

Toppings (your choice of . . .)

pepperoni slices, chopped onions, sliced mushrooms, sliced black olives, sliced jalapeños ("nacho slices"), sliced green peppers, pineapple chunks, Italian sausage, sliced tomatoes, sliced ham, anchovies

1. To prepare the crust, dissolve the yeast with the warm water in a small bowl or measuring cup and let it sit for 5 minutes.
2. Sift the flour, salt, and baking soda together in a large bowl.
3. Cut the shortening into the flour and mix the ingredients together with your hands until the shortening is reduced to tiny pea-size pieces.
4. Make an indention in the flour and pour in the milk and yeast mixture. Using a fork, stir the liquid around in the center, slowly drawing in more flour as you stir. When all of the flour is moistened and you can no longer stir with a fork, use your hands to combine the ingredients into a ball.
5. On a lightly floured surface, knead the dough with the heel of your hands. Continue kneading until the dough is smooth and silky, about 10 minutes.
6. Form the dough into a ball and put it into a large bowl covered with plastic wrap. Let the dough rise in a warm place for about 2 hours. After 2 hours, place the covered container into the refrigerator to rise overnight. Take the dough out of the refrigerator 2 hours before you plan to cook the pizza so that the dough can warm up to room temperature.

7. You may want to make the pizza sauce a day ahead as well, at the same time as you prepare the dough. Combine all of the ingredients in a small saucepan over medium heat until it bubbles. Reduce the heat and simmer for about 1 hour. When the sauce is cool, store it in the refrigerator.

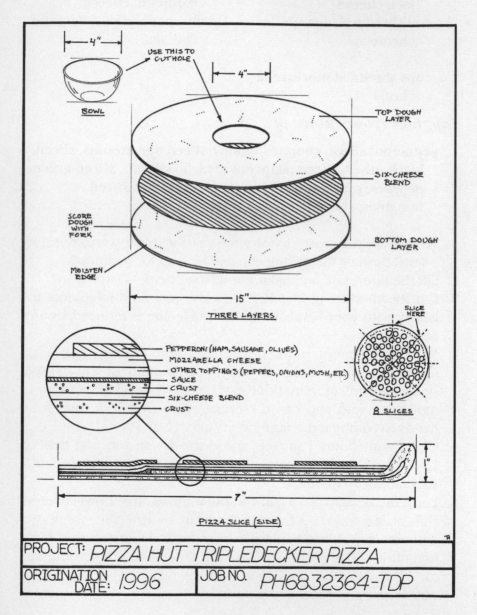

4"

USE THIS TO
CUT HOLE

4"

BOWL

TOP DOUGH
LAYER

SIX-CHEESE
BLEND

SCORE
DOUGH
WITH
FORK

BOTTOM DOUGH
LAYER

MOISTEN
EDGE

15"

THREE LAYERS

SLICE
HERE

PEPPERONI (HAM, SAUSAGE, OLIVES)
MOZZARELLA CHEESE
OTHER TOPPINGS (PEPPERS, ONIONS, MUSH., ETC.)
SAUCE
CRUST
SIX-CHEESE BLEND
CRUST

8 SLICES

1"

7"

PIZZA SLICE (SIDE)

PROJECT: PIZZA HUT TRIPLEDECKER PIZZA

ORIGINATION DATE: 1996   JOB NO. PH6832364-TDP

218

8. Preheat the oven to 475 degrees. Divide the dough in half, and form the two halves into balls. On a floured surface roll out each of the dough balls until they form thin 15-inch circles. Use a fork to poke the dough several times on the surface. This will keep the crust from bubbling. Place one of the crusts on a pizza pan that has been well-greased or sprinkled with cornmeal.

9. Combine the six cheeses to make the blend for the second layer. Sprinkle the cheese blend evenly over the pizza crust in the pan. Leave about a half-inch margin around the outside edge of the dough. Moisten the dough by brushing some water around the outside edge in that margin.

10. While the top pizza dough sits on a hard, floured surface, use an inverted bowl with a 4-inch diameter as a guide to cut a 4-inch circle out of the center of the dough. This is to keep the crusts from separating at the tip of each pizza slice when cut. Carefully place the dough on top of the cheese layer and crimp the edges together. Bend the crust up to form a lip. Brush some olive oil just on that lip all of the way around the pizza.

11. Spread the pizza sauce over the surface of the top pizza dough layer to the lip around the edge.

12. Sprinkle any vegetable toppings (or pineapple) on the pizza sauce. Sprinkle the 1½ cups mozzarella cheese over the pizza to the lip around the edge. Place any meat toppings or the olives on top of the cheese.

13. Bake the pizza for 12 to 15 minutes.

14. Slice the pizza 4 times through the center, making 8 slices.

✳ Planet Hollywood Pizza Bread

Serves 2 to 4 as an appetizer

Menu Description: "Fresh baked on premises, sliced into eight pieces, brushed with garlic butter, Parmesan cheese, mozzarella and basil, topped with chopped plum tomatoes and herbed olive oil."

In 1988, London-born restaurant mogul Robert Ian Earl joined with movie producer Keith Barrish and a gaggle of celebrities including Arnold Schwarzenegger, Sylvester Stallone, Bruce Willis, and Demi Moore to start a Hollywood-themed restaurant that is on its way to becoming his most successful venture yet. In 1991, a gala star-studded affair in New York City celebrated the opening of the world's first Planet Hollywood.

But even the coolest theme restaurant won't fly if the food doesn't please. Earl told *Nation's Restaurant News*, "People don't eat themes—no concept in the world can succeed for long unless it also delivers great food at the right price." So Planet Hollywood has created a menu of delicious dishes rivaling food from national chains that don't have a theme to lean on.

The Pizza Bread appetizer comes highly recommended by Planet Hollywood servers. The "bread" is actually just pizza dough, rolled thin, with a light layer of cheese, basil, and tomato on top; then it's baked in a special pizza oven at the restaurant. Since most of us don't have these ovens at home, this recipe has been designed for a conventional gas or electric oven.

1 12-inch thin-crust uncooked pizza dough (see Tidbits)	2 tablespoons coarsely chopped fresh basil
½ teaspoon garlic salt	1 small tomato, chopped (use a Roma or plum tomato if available)
1½ tablespoons butter, melted	
1 cup shredded mozzarella cheese	2 tablespoons grated Parmesan cheese

1. Preheat the oven to 475 degrees F.
2. If you are making your own crust, roll out the dough to a 12-inch diameter.
3. Mix the garlic salt with the butter.
4. Use a brush to coat the entire crust with garlic butter.
5. Spread half of the mozzarella cheese over the crust.

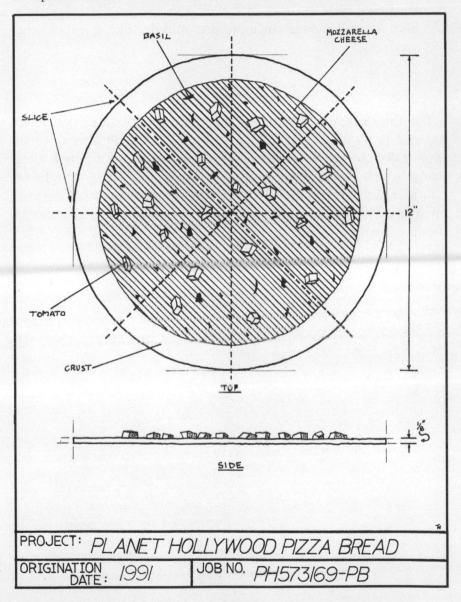

BASIL

MOZZARELLA CHEESE

SLICE

TOMATO

CRUST

TOP

12"

SIDE

⅛"

PROJECT: *PLANET HOLLYWOOD PIZZA BREAD*

ORIGINATION DATE: *1991*

JOB NO. *PH573169-PB*

6. Spread the basil over the cheese.
7. Spread the remaining mozzarella over the basil.
8. Sprinkle the tomato over the cheese.
9. Bake for 8 to 10 minutes or until the surface begins to turn brown.
10. Remove the pizza bread from the oven and sprinkle the fresh Parmesan over it.
11. Slice into 8 pieces through the middle, like a pizza, and serve hot.

Tidbits

For the dough you can use the recipe for pizza dough from page 62, or a canned tube of pizza dough (such as Pillsbury), or an instant dough mix. You will need only about 1 cup of dough after rising, which is about half a tube of the Pillsbury-type dough. Of course, I highly recommend making the dough from scratch if you have time. There's nothing in a box or can that tastes as good as the homemade stuff.

* Planet Hollywood Chicken Crunch

Serves 2 to 4 as an appetizer or snack

Menu Description: "A basket of tender chicken breaded with Cap'n Crunch and seasonings, served with Creole mustard sauce."

The Orlando, Florida Planet Hollywood, which had its big opening in 1994, pulls in yearly sales receipts totaling around $50 million, making it the highest volume restaurant in America. If you've never tried the Chicken Crunch at Planet Hollywood, you're missing a treat. Sliced chicken breast fingers are coated with a crunchy, slightly sweet breading combination of Cap'n Crunch cereal and cornflake crumbs. The chicken is then deep-fried to a golden brown and served with a tasty dipping sauce made from mayonnaise, horseradish, and Dijon mustard. You've probably tasted nothing like it.

Creole Mustard Sauce

2 tablespoons Grey
   Poupon Country Dijon
   mustard
3 tablespoons mayonnaise

1 teaspoon yellow mustard
1 teaspoon cream-style
   horseradish
1 teaspoon honey

Vegetable oil for frying
2 boneless, skinless chicken
   breast halves
2 cups Cap'n Crunch cereal
½ cup cornflake crumbs
½ teaspoon onion powder

½ teaspoon garlic powder
½ teaspoon salt
¼ teaspoon white pepper
1 egg, beaten
1 cup milk

1. Preheat oil in a deep pan or deep fryer to 375 degrees F. You want to use enough oil to completely cover the chicken 1 to 2 inches deep.
2. Combine all of the ingredients for the Creole mustard sauce in a small bowl and chill the sauce while the chicken is prepared.

223

3. Cut each chicken breast, lengthwise, into 5 long slices (chicken fingers).
4. Smash the Cap'n Crunch into crumbs using a food processor, or put the cereal into a plastic bag and start pounding.
5. Combine the cereals, onion powder, garlic powder, salt, and pepper in a medium bowl.

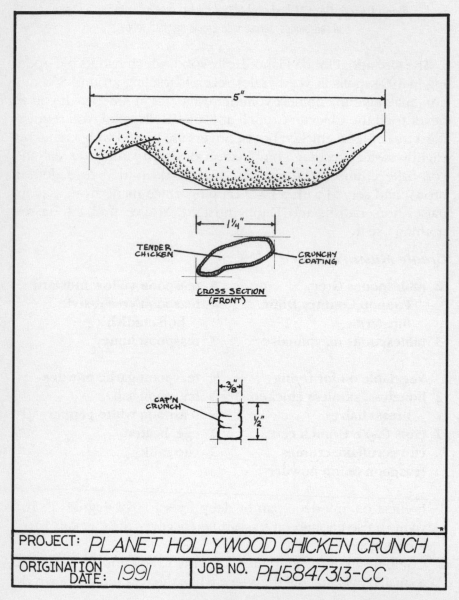

PROJECT: PLANET HOLLYWOOD CHICKEN CRUNCH

ORIGINATION DATE: 1991   JOB NO. PH5847313-CC

6. Combine the egg with the milk in a separate bowl.
7. Dredge each piece of chicken in the milk mixture, then completely coat it with the dry mixture. Do this for all the chicken before frying.
8. When the oil is hot, fry the chicken for 4 to 6 minutes or until golden to dark brown and crispy. Remove to paper towels or a rack to drain. Serve hot with Creole mustard sauce on the side for dipping.

✳ Planet Hollywood Pot Stickers

Serves 3 to 6 as an appetizer or snack

Menu Description: "Six pot stickers filled with fresh ground turkey meat seasoned with ginger, water chestnuts, red pepper and green onions. They are fried and served in a basket with spicy hoisin."

Planet Hollywood is known for the film and television memorabilia displayed throughout the restaurants. Some of the items on display behind thick Plexiglas include the genie bottle from *I Dream of Jeannie,* Val Kilmer's bat suit from *Batman Forever,* Tom Hanks' costume from *Forrest Gump,* Judy Garland's dress from *The Wizard of Oz,* and the painting from the set of the television show *Friends.* In addition to the memorabilia is a wall at the entrance to each restaurant that displays handprints in plaster from the likes of Mel Gibson, Jimmy Stewart, Harrison Ford, Demi Moore, Samuel L. Jackson, Paul Newman, Goldie Hawn, Patrick Swayze, and many others.

Pot stickers are a popular Asian dumpling that can be fried, steamed, or simmered in a broth. Planet Hollywood has customized its version to make them crunchier than the traditional dish, and it's a tasty twist. Since hoisin sauce would be very difficult to make from scratch, you can use a commercial brand found in most stores.

¼ **pound ground turkey**
½ **teaspoon minced fresh ginger**
1 **teaspoon minced green onion**
1 **teaspoon minced water chestnuts**
½ **teaspoon soy sauce**
½ **teaspoon ground black pepper**

¼ **teaspoon crushed red pepper flakes (no seeds)**
¼ **teaspoon salt**
⅛ **teaspoon garlic powder**
1 **egg, beaten**
Vegetable oil for frying
12 **wonton wrappers (3 × 3-inch size)**

On the Side

Hoisin sauce

1. In a small bowl, combine all the ingredients except the egg, wrappers, and oil. Add 1 tablespoon of the beaten egg. Save the rest of the egg for later. Preheat oil in a deep fryer or a deep saucepan to 375 degrees F. Use enough oil to cover the pot stickers—1 to 2 inches should be enough.

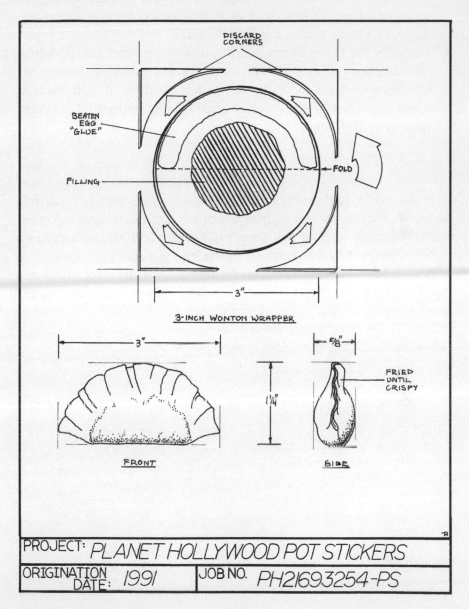

DISCARD CORNERS

BEATEN EGG "GLUE"

FILLING

FOLD

3"

3-INCH WONTON WRAPPER

3"

5/8"

1 1/4"

FRIED UNTIL CRISPY

FRONT

SIDE

PROJECT: PLANET HOLLYWOOD POT STICKERS

ORIGINATION DATE: 1991

JOB NO. PH21693254-PS

2. Invert a small bowl or glass with a 3-inch diameter on the center of a wonton wrapper and cut around it to make a circle. Repeat for the remaining wrappers.
3. Spoon ½ tablespoon of the turkey filling into the center of one wrapper. Brush a little beaten egg around half of the edge of the wrapper and fold the wrapper over the filling. Gather the wrapper as you seal it, so that it is crinkled around the edge. Repeat with the remaining ingredients.
4. Deep-fry the pot stickers, six at a time, in the hot oil for 3 to 6 minutes or until they are brown. Drain on a rack or paper towels. Serve with the hoisin sauce for dipping. If you want a spicier sauce, add some more crushed red pepper or cayenne pepper to the sauce.

Tidbits

If you can't find wonton wrappers, you can also use eggroll wrappers for this recipe. Eggroll wrappers are much bigger, so you will be wasting more of the dough when you trim the wrappers to 3-inch-diameter circles. But in a pinch, this is a quick solution.

Pot sticker wrappers can also be found in some supermarkets, but I've found the wonton wrappers and eggroll wrappers, when fried, taste more like the restaurant version.

✳ Red Lobster
Broiled Lobster

Serves 2 as an entree

The namesake of the Red Lobster chain is the delicious broiled lobster, lightly seasoned, served with lemon and melted butter. Two varieties are most often available at the restaurant: Maine lobster and rock lobster. The Maine lobsters are purchased live, while rock lobster tails come frozen; and both are available in stores across the country. Rock lobsters, also known as spiny lobsters, are found in warmer waters. They have no claws, which is why you only get rock lobster tails. Each Red Lobster restaurant has a special device that bakes and broils the lobsters without burning them. Since these special broilers don't come with most homes, I've created a cooking method using a conventional oven that produces broiled lobster just like that which you can enjoy at the restaurant.

2 6-ounce rock lobster or Maine lobster tails	Dash ground black pepper
Melted butter	Dash cayenne pepper
¼ teaspoon salt	Dash allspice
¼ teaspoon paprika	Lemon wedges

1. Thaw lobster tails if frozen, then preheat the oven to 425 degrees F.
2. Each tail is prepared differently for cooking. The meat from the rock lobster is fully exposed on top of the shell for broiling, while the meat of the Maine lobster is left in the shell.

    To prepare the rock lobster, use a kitchen scissors to cut along the top of the shell down to the tail. Crack the ribs of the shell underneath so that you can spread the shell open on top and pull the meat out down to the tail. You may have to use a spoon to pull the meat away from inside of the shell so that it will come free. Leave the end of the meat attached to the shell when you pull it out, then close the shell underneath it. Now

229

you should be able to rest the meat back down on top of the shell. Cut about ¼ inch deep down the center of the meat so that you can pull the colored part of the meat over, exposing the white center. This may have already happened when you cut the shell open.

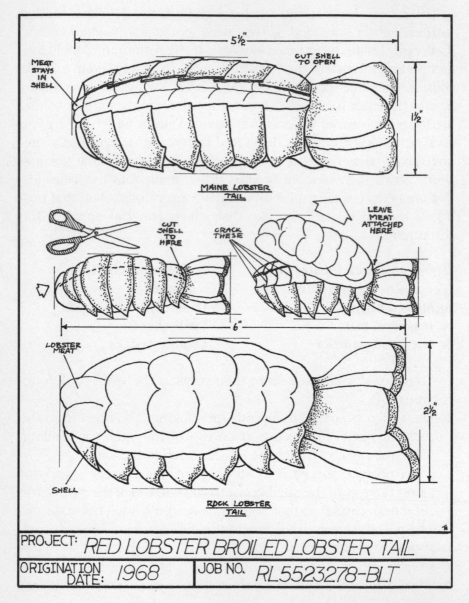

5½"

MEAT STAYS IN SHELL

CUT SHELL TO OPEN

1½"

MAINE LOBSTER TAIL

CUT SHELL TO HERE

CRACK THESE

LEAVE MEAT ATTACHED HERE

6"

LOBSTER MEAT

2½"

SHELL

ROCK LOBSTER TAIL

PROJECT: RED LOBSTER BROILED LOBSTER TAIL

ORIGINATION DATE: 1968

JOB NO. RL5523278-BLT

For the Maine lobster, slice down the top of the shell to the tail. Crack the ribs in the center along the bottom of the tail so that you can hinge the shell open from the top. Use a spoon to pull the meat away from the inside of the shell so that it is easy to eat when cooked, but leave the meat inside the shell. Slice down the middle of the meat so that you can spread open the colored part. This may have already happened when you cut the top of the shell open.

3. Brush the lobster meat with melted butter.
4. Combine the salt, paprika, peppers, and allspice in a small bowl. Sprinkle a dash of this spice combination on the top of each lobster.
5. Bake in the oven on a broiling pan for 15 minutes.
6. Turn the oven to broil and broil for an additional 6 to 8 minutes or until the meat or shell just begins to turn a light brown on top. Be careful not to burn the lobster meat. Remove from the broiler and serve with melted butter and a lemon wedge.

Tidbits

If you like, you can take the Maine lobster meat out of the shell as explained in the method for the rock lobster. That's not the way Red Lobster docs it, but, hey, you're not eating at Red Lobster.

✴ Red Lobster Scallops and Bacon

At the time I was researching this book there were two ways you could have your bacon and scallops at Red Lobster: wrapped and broiled, or grilled on a skewer. The former is a smaller portion to be served as an appetizer, while the skewers may be served as a main entree or part of one. I've included recipes to clone both versions.

✴ Broiled Bacon-Wrapped Scallops

Serves 2 as an appetizer

4	medium sea scallops	Ground pepper
2	slices bacon	1 tablespoon warm bottled
	Melted butter	clam juice
	Salt	4 toothpicks
	Paprika	

1. Preheat the broiler to high.
2. Boil 2 to 3 cups of water in a small pan over high heat. Salt the water.
3. Boil the scallops in the water for 3 to 4 minutes, or until they firm up. Drain the scallops when they're done.
4. Cook the bacon slices for a couple minutes per side. Don't cook until crispy or you won't be able to fold the bacon around the scallops.
5. When the scallops are cool enough to touch, cut or tear a piece of partially cooked bacon in half and wrap one half over the top of the scallop so that it meets itself underneath. Put a toothpick through the bacon to stick it in place. If you have a problem wrapping your bacon (story of my life) because it is too crispy, dip the bacon into hot or boiling water to make it more flexible. Repeat this with the remaining scallops.

6. Put the scallops on their side in an oven-safe dish and brush with melted butter.
7. Lightly season the scallops with salt, paprika, and a dash of ground pepper.
8. Broil the scallops for 5 to 6 minutes, or just until the edges begin to brown.
9. Remove the scallops from the oven and add warm clam juice to the bottom of the baking dish. Serve in the same dish.

✳ Grilled Scallop and Bacon Skewers

Serves 2 as an entree

1 teaspoon salt	2 slices bacon, cooked soft
16 sea scallops	1 tablespoon melted
4 round zucchini slices,	butter
½ inch thick	4 8-inch skewers

On the Side

Brown rice

1. Preheat the barbecue grill to medium/high heat.
2. In a large saucepan, heat 3 to 4 cups of water until boiling. Add a teaspoon or so of salt to the water.
3. Boil the scallops for 4 minutes or until they firm up.
4. Remove the scallops from the water and drain.
5. When the scallops have cooled enough to handle, begin building your 4 skewers.
6. Cut a zucchini slice in half and pierce it, round edge first, onto the skewer.
7. Slide the zucchini to the end until there's about 1 inch left on the end of the skewer.
8. Slide one scallop on next, piercing through the rounded edges.

233

9. Break the bacon into quarters and slide one piece of bacon on next.
10. Add two more scallops, one more piece of bacon, another scallop, and the other half of the zucchini slice (this one goes cut side first).
11. Make three more skewers exactly the same way.

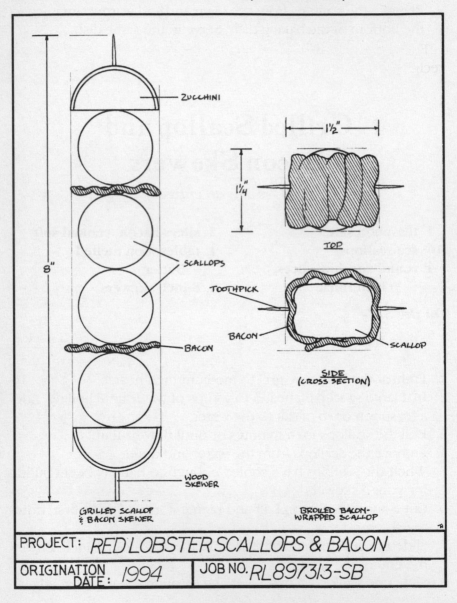

ZUCCHINI

SCALLOPS

BACON

WOOD SKEWER

8"

GRILLED SCALLOP & BACON SKEWER

1½"

1¼"

TOP

TOOTHPICK

BACON

SCALLOP

SIDE
(CROSS SECTION)

BROILED BACON-WRAPPED SCALLOP

PROJECT: *RED LOBSTER SCALLOPS & BACON*

ORIGINATION DATE: *1994*

JOB NO. *RL 897313-SB*

12. Generously brush the skewers with melted butter.
13. Lightly season with salt, paprika, and a dash of black pepper.
14. Grill the skewers for 4 to 5 minutes per side or until the zucchini has softened. Serve the skewers over a bed of brown rice.

Tidbits

For a healthier alternative, try turkey bacon with either of these recipes as a substitute for the pork bacon.

✳ Red Lobster Stuffed Shrimp and Stuffed Mushrooms

Serves 4 to 6 as an appetizer

Bill Darden was only 19 when he started his restaurant career in 1939 by opening a 25-seat lunch counter called The Green Frog in Waycross, Georgia. From the start Bill's business was a hopping success. That success helped Bill to springboard into other restaurant acquisitions throughout the years including 20 Howard Johnson's restaurants. Then, in 1968, as he reached his mid-fifties, Bill took another gamble and opened a seafood restaurant in Lakeland, Florida. When deciding on a name for the new restaurant, someone suggested that since he had great luck with the name "Green Frog" in the past, why not name this one "Red Lobster." And so it was.

Here are a couple of great dishes to serve as appetizers or on the side with an entree such as broiled lobster or fish. These recipes include a stuffing that varies in the restaurants only in the type of seafood used—the stuffed shrimp contains crabmeat and the stuffed mushrooms contain lobster meat. If you like, you can use the stuffings interchangeably in the mushrooms caps and shrimp.

✳ Stuffed Shrimp

½ cup water
3 tablespoons butter
1 tablespoon minced celery
1 tablespoon minced onion
1 tablespoon finely chopped
    red chili pepper

1 tablespoon finely chopped
    green chili pepper
¼ teaspoon dried parsley
½ teaspoon salt
Dash pepper
½ tablespoon sugar

236

¾ cup cornbread crumbs
   (Pepperidge Farm
   cornbread stuffing
   mix is good)
1 cup lump crab meat (fresh,
   frozen, or one 6-ounce can)

1 egg, beaten
20 large shrimp
¼ to ½ pound Cheddar
   cheese, thinly sliced
Paprika

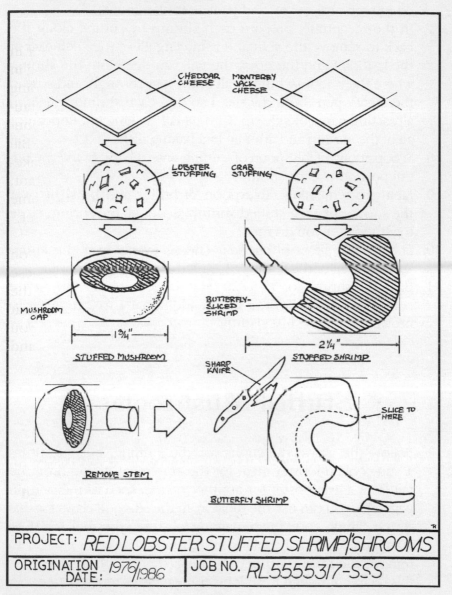

PROJECT: *RED LOBSTER STUFFED SHRIMP/SHROOMS*

ORIGINATION DATE: 1976/1986   JOB NO. *RL5555317-SSS*

1. Preheat the oven to 375 degrees F.
2. Boil the water and 2 tablespoons butter in a medium saucepan.
3. Add the celery, onion, peppers, parsley, salt, pepper, and sugar.
4. Reduce the heat to low and let it simmer for 5 minutes.
5. Add the bread crumbs and remove from the heat.
6. Mix the crab meat with the beaten egg. Add to the bread-crumb mixture, cover, and let it sit for 5 minutes.
7. In the meantime, prepare each shrimp by cutting along the back to remove the vein and removing all of the shell except the last joint and the tip of the tail. Cut deep into the shrimp where the vein was, but not all of the way through, and spread the meat open (butterfly slice) so that each shrimp will sit in a roasting pan, cut side up, with its tail sticking up. Repeat for all of the shrimp and arrange in a baking dish.
8. Scoop about 1 tablespoon of stuffing onto the top of the spread-out portion of each shrimp.
9. Melt the remaining tablespoon of butter and brush it over the surface of each stuffed shrimp. Scoot all the shrimp close together after you do this.
10. Spread thin slices of cheddar cheese evenly over the entire surface of all of the shrimp. Sprinkle on a dash of paprika.
11. Bake the shrimp for 15 to 20 minutes or until the shrimp are completely cooked. Broil for an additional 1 to 2 minutes to brown the cheese just slightly.

✳ Stuffed Mushrooms

1. Follow the above directions for the stuffing, but substitute 1 cup cooked lobster meat for the crab meat. If you broil the tail from a live lobster for another recipe, such as the one on page 229, you can use the meat from the legs and claws for this recipe. Simply cook the remaining lobster in the shell for 15 to 20 minutes in rapidly boiling salted water. Use a nut cracker to remove the meat. You may also use canned lobster meat for this recipe, although fresh lobster meat tastes much better.

2. Instead of shrimp, use 20 to 24 (about 1 pound) mushrooms with stems removed.
3. Fill the mushroom caps with 2 to 3 teaspoons of stuffing, brush with melted butter, and top with slices of Monterey Jack cheese rather than Cheddar.
4. Season lightly with paprika, then bake the mushrooms in a roasting pan or baking dish in a preheated oven set on 375 degrees F for about 12 minutes, or until the cheese is melted. Broil for 1 to 2 minutes to slightly brown the cheese.

✳ Red Robin
No-Fire Peppers

Serves 2 to 4 as an appetizer

Menu Description: "Full-flavored jalapeños stuffed with cool
cream cheese and deep-fried in a cracker-crumb coating.
Served with sweet jalapeño jelly & sour cream."

Red Robin was one of the first restaurant chains to serve No-Fire
Peppers, an item which can be found on many restaurant menus
today under a variety of different names. The cream cheese–filled,
battered and fried jalapeño peppers are actually called Poppers by
their creators, Anchor Foods, a restaurant food supply company
which manufactures Poppers and a variety of other appetizers for
sale to restaurant chains everywhere. According to *Restaurants
and Institutions* magazine, Poppers were the #1 food item added
to restaurant menus in 1995, with restaurants purchasing over 700
million of the little suckers.

It's important when you make these that you allow time for
them to freeze. The freezing stage ensures that the coating stays
on when the peppers are fried and prevents the cream cheese
from squirting out as it heats up.

4 large, fresh jalapeño peppers	⅔ cup self-rising flour
¼ pound cream cheese	⅛ teaspoon garlic powder
2 eggs	Dash paprika
¾ teaspoon salt	Dash onion powder
1 teaspoon vegetable oil	½ cup cornflake crumbs
	Vegetable oil for frying

On the Side

Hot pepper jelly	Sour cream

1. Remove the stems from the jalapeños, then slice each one
   down the middle lengthwise and remove the seeds and inner
   membranes. Be careful to wash your hands afterward.

2. Poach the jalapeño halves in a saucepan half-filled with boiling water for 10 to 15 minutes or until tender. Drain and cool.
3. Blot with a cloth or paper towel to dry the inside of each jalapeño slice, then use a teaspoon to spread about ½ ounce of cream cheese into each jalapeño half.

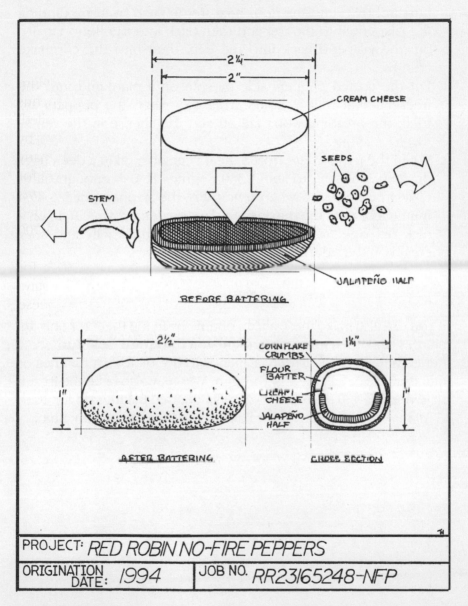

BEFORE BATTERING

AFTER BATTERING

CROSS SECTION

PROJECT: *RED ROBIN NO-FIRE PEPPERS*

ORIGINATION DATE: *1994* JOB NO. *RR23165248-NFP*

4. Beat the eggs in a small, shallow bowl, then add ¼ teaspoon salt and the oil and combine with a whisk.
5. In another shallow bowl, combine the flour, ½ teaspoon salt, garlic powder, paprika, and onion powder.
6. Add the cornflake crumbs to a third shallow bowl.
7. Working one at a time, dip each stuffed jalapeño into the egg mixture, then into the flour mixture. Repeat, by again dipping the jalapeño into the egg and then back into the flour. Finally, dip the jalapeño back into the egg, then into the cornflake crumbs.
8. Put the coated peppers side by side on a plate and into the freezer for at least 2 hours. This way when the peppers are fried, the breading won't fall off and the cheese in the center won't ooze out.
9. When the peppers are frozen, heat vegetable oil in a deep fryer or deep saucepan to about 350 degrees F. Use enough oil to cover the jalapeños when frying. Fry the peppers for 3½ to 4 minutes or until the outside is a dark golden brown. Drain on a rack or paper towels. Serve hot with pepper jelly and sour cream on the side.

Tidbits

You can also make these ahead of time by frying them for only 1½ minutes and then refreezing them until you are ready to serve them. Then cook the frozen jalapeños in hot oil for 3½ minutes or until they are hot all the way through. You may also bake the frozen jalapeños in a 450 degrees F oven on a greased baking pan for 10 to 15 minutes, turning them over halfway through the heating time.

✳ Red Robin
BBQ Chicken Salad

Serves 1 as an entree (can be doubled)

Menu Description: "Breast of chicken basted with BBQ sauce & topped with cheddar cheese, tomato, fresh avocado, and black beans. Served with Ranch dressing & garlic cheese bread."

In 1969, Gerald Kingen bought a beat-up 30-year-old bar called Red Robin in Seattle across the road from the University of Washington. The pub did a booming business with the college and local crowd, but in 1973 building officials gave their opinion of the bar: Either fix it up or shut it down. Jerry not only fixed up the 1200-square-foot building, but also expanded it to three times its old size, to 3600 square feet, and added a kitchen to start making food. Red Robin soon became popular for its wide selection of gourmet burgers in addition to the designer cocktails served in kooky glasses. Jerry says he set out to create a chain of restaurants that would be recognized as "the adult McDonald's and poor man's Trader Vic's."

2 cups chopped romaine lettuce

2 cups chopped green leaf or iceberg lettuce

½ cup chopped red cabbage

1 small tomato, chopped (¼ cup)

1 boneless, skinless chicken breast half

⅓ cup barbecue sauce (Bullseye or K.C. Masterpiece work well)

½ cup canned refried black beans

½ cup shredded Cheddar cheese

¼ cup French's French Fried Onions (onion straws)

3 avocado slices (¼ avocado)

¼ cup ranch dressing

1. Toss the lettuces and cabbage together and arrange on a large plate.

243

2. Arrange the tomato on the lettuce mixture at the bottom of the plate.
3. Grill the chicken breast on a hot barbecue grill for 4 to 5 minutes per side or until done. Brush a generous coating of barbecue sauce over the chicken as it grills.

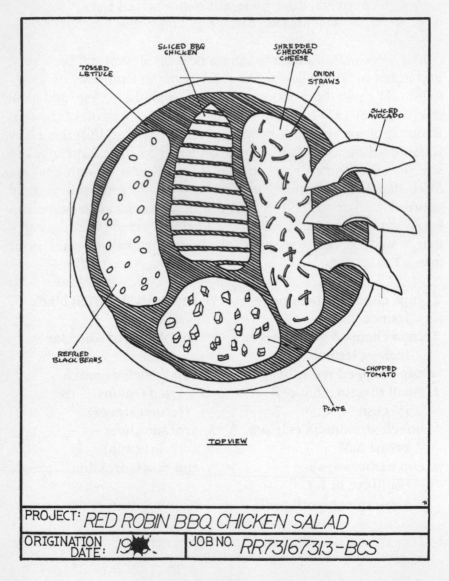

TOSSED LETTUCE

SLICED BBQ CHICKEN

SHREDDED CHEDDAR CHEESE

ONION STRAWS

SLICED AVOCADO

REFRIED BLACK BEANS

CHOPPED TOMATO

PLATE

TOP VIEW

PROJECT: *RED ROBIN BBQ CHICKEN SALAD*

ORIGINATION DATE: 19█.   JOB NO. *RR73167313-BCS*

4. Heat the black beans in the microwave or in a saucepan over medium heat.
5. Spread the black beans over the lettuce on the left side of the plate.
6. Slice the warm chicken into bite-size pieces and arrange them neatly over the lettuce in the center of the plate.
7. Sprinkle the cheese over the lettuce on the right side of the plate.
8. Sprinkle the onion straws over the cheese.
9. Garnish the salad with 3 slices of avocado arranged side by side on the right rim of the plate. Serve with the ranch dressing and the remaining barbecue sauce on the side.

Tidbits

You can also make the onion straws yourself by following this simple recipe:

Onion Straws

2 cups vegetable oil	½ teaspoon baking soda
¼ cup very thinly sliced white onion	¼ teaspoon salt
	⅔ cup cold water
½ cup all-purpose flour	

1. Heat the oil in a wide saucepan to about 350 degrees F.
2. Slice the onion into very thin onion rings and then cut the rings in half, making long strips or straws. Try to slice the onion as thin as possible.
3. Combine the flour, baking soda, and salt in a large bowl. Add the cold water and whisk until the batter is smooth.
4. When the oil is hot, drop the onions into the batter. Remove the onions one at a time, let them drip off a bit, and then place them into the hot oil. You will want to cook these for about 2 minutes apiece, or until you see them turn a golden brown. Drain the onion straws on a paper towel.

✳ Red Robin
Mountain High Mudd Pie

Serves 12

Gerald Kingen is a man with a mission. In 1985 he sold his successful Red Robin chain of restaurants to Tokyo-based Skylark Co. Ltd. Unhappy with the changes the new owners were implementing, Jerry and a partner purchased a "substantial equity position" of the Irvine, California–based Red Robin in March of 1996. Now Jerry is once again at the helm of the company, with a goal of reviving old menu items and living up to the old slogan as "the world's greatest gourmet burger maker & most masterful mixologists."

A unique signature dessert item is the Mountain High Mudd Pie, which servers claim is one of the most ordered desserts on the menu. Save some room for this giant-size sundae made from chocolate and vanilla ice cream with peanut butter, caramel, and fudge sauce. There are several stages of freezing, so give yourself at least seven hours to allow for these steps. This dessert is big and serves at least a dozen, so it's good for a small party or gathering, or makes a unique birthday cake. If there's only a few of you, leftovers can be frozen in a sealed container for several weeks and enjoyed later.

6 cups chocolate ice cream	1 20-ounce squirt bottle chocolate topping
1 cup peanut butter cookie pieces	1 20-ounce squirt bottle caramel topping
6 cups vanilla ice cream	1 can whipped cream
1⅔ cups creamy peanut butter	¾ cup chopped peanuts
4 chocolate-flavored graham crackers	12 maraschino cherries, with stems
1 cup fudge topping	

1. Soften the chocolate ice cream and load it into the bottom of a 2½- to 3-quart mixing bowl. Make sure the surface of the ice cream is smooth and leveled.
2. Spread the peanut butter cookie pieces evenly over the top of

the ice cream, then cover the bowl and put it back into the freezer for at least 1 hour. (If you can't find packaged peanut butter cookies, use the recipe in "Tidbits.")

3. Soften the vanilla ice cream and spread it over the chocolate ice cream and cookie pieces. Again, be sure to smooth and level the surface of the ice cream. Cover the bowl with plastic wrap and put it back into the freezer for at least 1 hour.

4. Use a spatula to spread ⅔ cup of peanut butter over the surface of the ice cream. Be sure the ice cream has hardened before you do this or it could get sloppy.

5. Crush the chocolate graham crackers into crumbs and spread them evenly over the peanut butter. Put the bowl back into the freezer for at least 1 hour.

6. Remove the bowl from the freezer and hold it in a sink filled with warm water for about 1 minute. You want the ice cream around the edges to soften just enough that you can invert the ice cream onto a plate.

7. Turn a large plate upside down and place it on top of the bowl. Flip the bowl and plate over together, and tap gently on the bowl until the ice cream falls out onto the plate. You may have to put the bowl back into the water if it's stubborn. Once the ice cream is out, cover it with plastic wrap and place it back in the freezer for another 1 or 2 hours.

8. Without heating it up, spread the fudge evenly over the entire surface of the ice cream mountain. Put the fudge-coated ice cream back into the freezer for 1 hour.

9. When the fudge has hardened, spread the remaining 1 cup of peanut butter over the entire surface as well. Once again, back into the freezer for at least 1 hour. We're almost there.

10. Slice the ice cream with a warm knife into 12 pieces. Put wax paper between the cuts so that when you serve it later, it is easy to divide. Then slip it back into the freezer, covered.

11. When serving, first coat a plate with a criss-cross pattern of chocolate and caramel sauce. Make three parallel lines down the plate with the squirt bottle of chocolate sauce. Then three parallel horizontal lines made with the bottle of caramel sauce.

12. Place the slice of ice cream upright onto the plate toward the back of the design.

247

13. Spray whipped cream on top and down the curved edge of the ice cream slice, onto the plate over the sauces. Be generous.
14. Sprinkle about a tablespoon of chopped nuts over your creation.
15. Add a cherry to the top. Marvel at the beauty, then dig in or serve it before it melts. Repeat for the remaining slices.

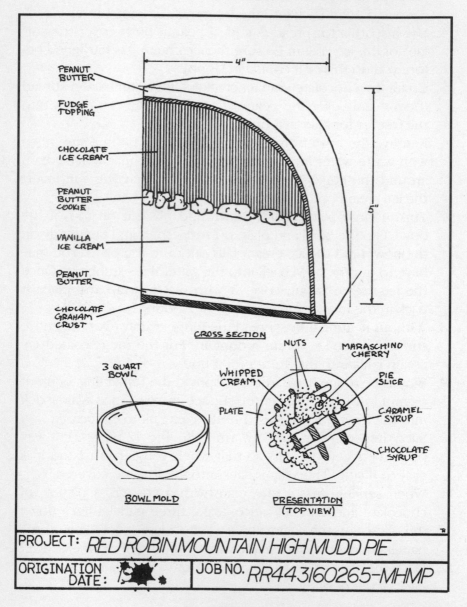

PEANUT BUTTER

FUDGE TOPPING

CHOCOLATE ICE CREAM

PEANUT BUTTER COOKIE

VANILLA ICE CREAM

PEANUT BUTTER

CHOCOLATE GRAHAM CRUST

4"

5"

CROSS SECTION

3 QUART BOWL

WHIPPED CREAM

PLATE

NUTS

MARASCHINO CHERRY

PIE SLICE

CARAMEL SYRUP

CHOCOLATE SYRUP

BOWL MOLD

PRESENTATION (TOP VIEW)

PROJECT: RED ROBIN MOUNTAIN HIGH MUDD PIE

ORIGINATION DATE:

JOB NO. RR443160265-MHMP

Tidbits

If you would like to make your own peanut butter cookies, rather than buying them pre-made, here is a recipe that makes about 2 dozen tasty cookies—more than enough for the ice cream dessert.

Peanut Butter Cookies

½ cup butter, softened
½ cup granulated sugar
½ cup firmly packed brown
   sugar
½ cup creamy peanut butter

1 egg
1¼ teaspoons vanilla extract
1½ cups all-purpose flour
1 teaspoon baking soda
½ teaspoon salt

1. Preheat the oven to 325 degrees F.
2. Use an electric mixer to combine the butter with the sugars in a large bowl until creamy.
3. Add the peanut butter, egg, and vanilla and mix until smooth.
4. Sift together the flour, baking soda, and salt, and combine with the moist ingredients in the large bowl. Mix the dough until all of the ingredients are smooth and well blended.
5. Drop rounded tablespoons of the dough onto an ungreased cookie sheet. Press the dough flat with a fork and bake for 15 to 18 minutes, until the edges of the cookies begin to turn light brown.

✳ Ruby Tuesday Potato Cheese Soup

Serves 4 as an appetizer, 2 as an entree

Sandy Beall started managing Pizza Huts while a freshman at the University of Tennessee, to get out of fraternity house duties. It was just three years later that Sandy's boss at Pizza Hut would favor him with quite a nice gift: $10,000 to invest in a dream. With that, Sandy and four of his fraternity buddies pitched in to open the first Ruby Tuesday on the university campus in Knoxville, Tennessee, in 1972. Sandy was only 21 at the time.

Here's a great soup that can be served by the cup or in large bowls as a meal in itself. Along with the potatoes is a little bit of minced celery, some minced onion, and a small amount of grated carrot for color. An additional pinch of cheese, crumbled bacon, and chopped green onion make a tasty garnish just like on the Ruby Tuesday original.

2 **large russet potatoes**	2 **tablespoons flour**
2 **tablespoons finely minced celery (½ stalk)**	1½ **cups milk**
1 **tablespoon finely minced onion**	1 **cup plus 1 tablespoon shredded Cheddar cheese**
1 **tablespoon grated carrot (¼ carrot)**	1 **tablespoon shredded Monterey Jack cheese**
2 **cups chicken stock or broth**	2 **slices bacon, cooked**
1 **teaspoon salt**	1 **tablespoon chopped green onion**
2 **teaspoons white vinegar**	

1. Peel the potatoes and chop them into bite-size pieces—you should have about 4 cups. Make sure the celery and onion are minced into very small pieces about the size of a grain of rice. The carrot should be grated into very small pieces, not shredded.
2. Combine the vegetables with the chicken stock, salt, and vinegar in a large saucepan over medium heat. Bring the stock to a boil, then turn down the heat, cover the pan, and simmer for 20 minutes.

3. Whisk together the flour and milk in a medium bowl.
4. Remove the saucepan of vegetables from the heat and add the flour and milk mixture. Put the pan back on the heat and simmer, uncovered, for 5 to 8 minutes or until the soup has thickened.
5. Add 1 cup Cheddar cheese to the soup and simmer until melted. By this time the potatoes should be tender and falling apart. If not, continue to cook until the soup is as thick as you like it.
6. To serve, spoon the soup into bowls. Divide the remaining 1 tablespoon of Cheddar and the Monterey Jack and sprinkle on the soup. Crumble the bacon and sprinkle it evenly on top of the cheese. Top off each bowl of soup with chopped green onion.

✳ Ruby Tuesday
Smokey Mountain Chicken

Serves 2 as an entree

Menu Description: "Chicken breast topped with ham, barbecue sauce, tomatoes, scallions and cheese. Served with fries."

When the founder of Ruby Tuesday, Sandy Beall, was reviewing some early designs of printed materials for his planned restaurant, he saw that some of the art featured the faces of University of Tennessee students printed in red. At that moment Sandy knew he wanted to call the eatery "ruby something." Meanwhile, he and the four fraternity friends who joined him in the investment had been listening to lots of Rolling Stones music. One day when Sandy heard "Ruby Tuesday" come on the jukebox, he convinced his partners that they had finally found a name.

You may find a little something unusual in the name for this dish. Ruby Tuesday's menu became a victim of a common spelling error in the word "smoky." Apparently the dish is named after the Great Smoky Mountains that lie between North Carolina and Tennessee, but there's no "e" in that name or in the general spelling of the word "smoky." But, hey, what do you want: good spelling or good taste? And this dish, which combines chicken breast, ham and barbecue sauce, topped with tomatoes, scallions and cheese, tastes great no matter how you spell it. Thanks, Rubey Tuesday.

2 whole boneless chicken breasts (with skin)
Vegetable or olive oil
Salt
Pinch dried thyme
Pinch dried summer savory
4 slices deli-sliced smoked ham

2 tablespoons hickory smoke barbecue sauce (Bullseye is good)
2 slices provolone cheese
½ medium tomato, chopped (¼ cup)
1 green onion, chopped (2 tablespoons)

252

On the Side

French fries   **Rice**

1. Prepare the barbecue or preheat the stovetop grill.
2. Rub a little oil on the chicken, then sprinkle some salt, thyme, and savory on each chicken breast.

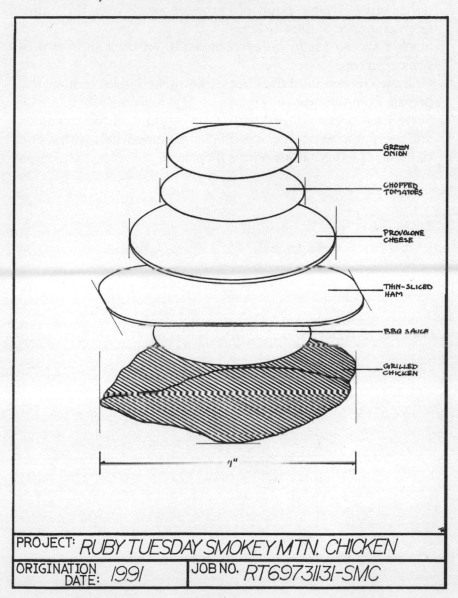

GREEN ONION

CHOPPED TOMATOES

PROVOLONE CHEESE

THIN-SLICED HAM

BBQ SAUCE

GRILLED CHICKEN

7"

PROJECT: *RUBY TUESDAY SMOKEY MTN. CHICKEN*

ORIGINATION DATE: *1991*   JOB NO. *RT6973II3I-SMC*

253

3. Grill the chicken on a hot, covered barbecue for 4 to 5 minutes per side, starting with the skin side up. When you flip the chicken over with the skin side down, wait a couple minutes, then put the slices of ham on the grill. This is just to heat up the ham; be careful not to scorch it.
4. When you think the chicken is about a minute away from being done, brush 1 tablespoon of barbecue sauce over the entire face-up surface of the chicken.
5. Stack 2 slices of ham on each breast, then lay a slice of provolone on top.
6. Grill the chicken until the cheese has melted, then remove the breasts from the heat.
7. Serve each breast topped with 2 tablespoons of the tomatoes and a tablespoon of green onion. Serve immediately with a side of French-fried potatoes or rice if desired.

✳ Ruby Tuesday
Sonora Chicken Pasta

Serves 4 as an entree

Menu Description: *"Penne pasta tossed in a spicy Southwestern cheese sauce, topped with grilled chicken, spicy black beans, scallions and more."*

If you like pasta, black beans, and chicken, you'll love having it all swimming together in this spicy cheese sauce. The chicken is prepared over an open grill, then sliced before laying it over a bed of pasta and cheese sauce. The black beans and peppers give this dish a decidedly Southwestern flair.

1 pound Velveeta cheese spread (or 1 16-ounce jar Cheez Whiz)	½ tablespoon vinegar
	¼ teaspoon cumin
	1 15-ounce can black beans
½ cup heavy cream	
2 tablespoons minced red chili pepper	Dash paprika
	4 boneless, skinless chicken breast halves
4 tablespoons green chili pepper (½ pepper), minced	Vegetable oil
	Dash dried thyme
4 tablespoons minced onion	Dash dried summer savory
1 clove garlic, minced	1 16-ounce box penne pasta
2 teaspoons olive oil	1 tablespoon butter
2 tablespoons water	2 Roma (plum) tomatoes, chopped
½ teaspoon salt	
2 teaspoons sugar	2 to 4 green onions, chopped

1. Prepare the barbecue or preheat your stovetop grill.
2. Combine the cheese spread with the cream in a small saucepan over medium/low heat. Stir the cheese often until it melts and becomes smooth.
3. Sauté the red chili pepper and 2 tablespoons green chili pepper, 2 tablespoons onion, and ½ clove garlic in the olive oil for a couple minutes then add the water to the pan so that the

255

peppers do not scorch. Simmer another 2 minutes or until the water has cooked off.

4. When the cheese is smooth, add the sautéed vegetables, ¼ teaspoon salt, sugar, vinegar, and cumin. Leave on low heat, stirring occasionally, until the other ingredients are ready.

5. Pour the entire can of beans with the liquid into a small saucepan over medium heat. Add the remaining green chili pepper, onions, garlic, a pinch of salt, and a dash of paprika. Bring the beans to a boil, stirring often, then reduce the heat to low and simmer until everything else is ready. By this time the beans will have thickened and the onions will have become transparent.

6. Rub the chicken breasts lightly with oil, then season with salt, thyme, and savory.

7. Cook the breasts on a hot grill for 5 minutes per side or until done. When they have cooked thoroughly, remove them from the grill and use a sharp knife to slice each breast into ½-inch slices, so that they are easier to eat. Retain the shape of the chicken breast by keeping the slices in order with one hand as you slice.

8. As the chicken cooks, prepare the pasta in a large pot filled with 3 to 4 quarts of boiling water. Cook the pasta for 12 to 14 minutes or until tender. Drain the pasta in a colander, and toss with the butter.

9. When everything is ready, spoon one-fourth of the pasta onto each plate.

10. Pour about ⅓ cup of cheese sauce over the pasta.

11. Carefully add a sliced breast of chicken, being sure to maintain its shape as you lay the slices on the bed of pasta.

12. Spread ⅓ cup of the black beans over the chicken.

13. Sprinkle ¼ cup of chopped tomatoes on the beans.

14. Sprinkle about 1 tablespoon of green onions on the tomatoes and serve immediately. Salt to taste.

Tidbits

You can make a lighter version of this meal by using the lower fat version of the Cheez Whiz or Velveeta cheese spreads.

* Ruby Tuesday
Strawberry Tallcake for Two

Makes six 2-person servings

Menu Description: "Three layers of light and airy sponge cake and strawberry mousse, drenched in strawberry sauce, topped with vanilla ice cream, fresh strawberries and whipped cream."

The Strawberry Tallcake is a signature, trademarked item for Ruby Tuesday. It's pretty big, so plan on sharing it. This copycat recipe requires that you bake the sponge cake in a large, shallow pan—I use a cookie sheet that has turned-up edges to hold in the batter. And you might find the strawberry mousse that is used to frost the cake makes a great, simple-to-make dessert on its own.

Strawberry Mousse and Sauce

1 10-ounce package frozen strawberries in syrup

1¾ cups water

1 3-ounce package strawberry Jell-O

1 cup heavy cream

Sponge Cake

5 eggs, separated

1½ cups sugar

½ cup cold water

2 teaspoons vanilla

1½ cups all-purpose flour

½ teaspoon baking powder

½ teaspoon salt

½ teaspoon cream of tartar

12 to 18 scoops vanilla ice cream (½ gallon)

½ pint fresh strawberries, sliced

1 can whipped cream

1. Defrost the frozen strawberries and pour the entire package, including the syrup, into a blender or food processor and purée for 10 to 15 seconds until smooth.
2. Combine the strawberry purée with 1½ cups of the water in a small saucepan over medium heat.
3. When the strawberry mixture comes to a boil, add the entire

257

package of Jell-O, stir to dissolve, and remove the pan from the heat to cool.

4. When the strawberry mixture has cooled to room temperature, divide it in half into two medium bowls.

5. Beat the whipping cream until it is thick and forms peaks. Fold the cream into one of the bowls of the strawberry mixture

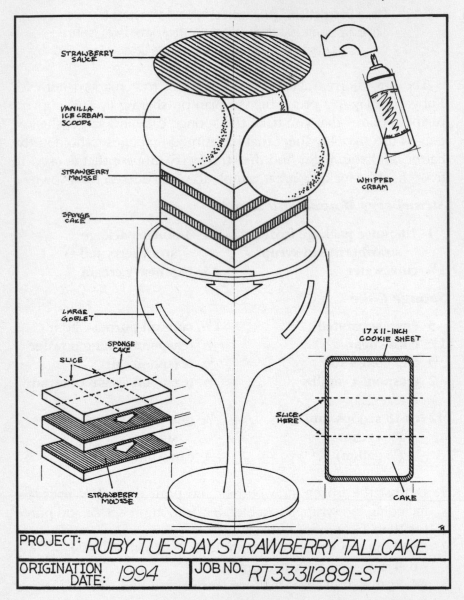

STRAWBERRY SAUCE

VANILLA ICE CREAM SCOOPS

STRAWBERRY MOUSSE

SPONGE CAKE

WHIPPED CREAM

LARGE GOBLET

SPONGE CAKE

SLICE

STRAWBERRY MOUSSE

17 X 11-INCH COOKIE SHEET

SLICE HERE

CAKE

PROJECT: RUBY TUESDAY STRAWBERRY TALLCAKE

ORIGINATION DATE: 1994

JOB NO. RT33112891-ST

until well combined. This is your strawberry mousse. Cover and chill.

6. To the other bowl, add the remaining ¼ cup of water. This is the strawberry syrup. Cover and chill this mixture as well.
7. Preheat the oven to 350 degrees F.
8. Beat the egg yolks until they turn creamy and a much lighter shade of yellow.
9. Add the sugar and blend it well into the yolks.
10. Add the water and vanilla and combine well with the yolks mixture.
11. Sift together the flour, baking powder, and salt, and add it to the yolk mixture. Mix well until the batter is smooth.
12. In a separate bowl, beat the egg whites until smooth, then add the cream of tartar. Continue beating until the whites are stiff and form peaks.
13. Fold the egg whites into the batter and mix slowly just until well combined.
14. Pour the batter into an ungreased 17 X 11-inch cookie sheet (with turned-up edges all the way around) and bake for 25 to 30 minutes or until the top of the sponge cake is a light brown color.
15. When the cake has cooled and the mousse has firmed up, you are ready to assemble the cake. First divide the cake into three even sections by cutting down the width of the cake twice with a sharp knife. Be sure the cake has come loose from the pan. You may need to use a spatula to unstick the cake sections.
16. Divide the mousse in half and spread each half onto two sections of the cake. Carefully place the layers on top of each other so that the mousse has been sandwiched in the middle between the three layers. This cake can be stored in the refrigerator for several days until you need it.
17. When you are ready to assemble the dessert, slice the cake into 6 even sections. Put a slice into a medium-sized bowl (or a large goblet if you have one), then arrange 2 to 3 scoops of vanilla ice cream around the cake. Pour a sixth (just over ¼ cup) of the strawberry sauce over the top of the cake and ice cream, sprinkle some sliced strawberries on top, then cover the thing with whipped cream. Repeat with the remaining servings.

✳ Ruth's Chris Steak House Barbecued Shrimp

Serves 2 as an appetizer

In 1965, Ruth Fertel, divorced with two kids in their teens, was looking for a better way to support herself in her native New Orleans. Her job as a lab technician wasn't paying enough for her to send the kids to college, so she went to the classifieds to find something better. There she found a steakhouse for sale, and determined that this might be her ticket. She mortgaged her house to raise $18,000 (against the advice of her attorney) and purchased the restaurant, then called Chris Steak House. Ruth sold 35 steaks on opening day—not much for a restaurant that now sells 10,000 a day. But the restaurant would eventually become a big hit, and within the first year Ruth was making more than twice her salary at the lab.

In keeping with the New Orleans flavor of many of the Ruth's Chris dishes, this barbecued shrimp is actually Cajun-style broiled shrimp with a little kick to it.

5 to 6 large uncooked shrimp
¼ cup (½ stick) butter, melted
1 tablespoon Louisiana hot sauce (Frank's Red Hot or Crystal are good)
2 cloves garlic, pressed
¼ teaspoon salt
½ teaspoon coarsely ground or cracked black pepper
½ teaspoon finely chopped fresh parsley
Pinch dried rosemary
Lemon wedges

1. Preheat the oven to 400 degrees F.
2. Shell and devein the shrimp.
3. In a small baking dish, combine the melted butter with the hot sauce, garlic, salt, cracked pepper, parsley, and rosemary. Stir.
4. Arrange the shrimp side by side in the baking dish and bake for 6 to 8 minutes. Immediately broil the shrimp for 2 to 4 minutes or until the shrimp are done, but not chewy. Squeeze some lemon juice over the shrimp. Serve the shrimp sizzling hot in the baking dish.

✳ Ruth's Chris Steak House Petite Filet

Serves 4 as an entree

Menu Description: "A smaller, but equally tender filet . . . the tenderest corn-fed Mid-western beef. So tender it practically melts in your mouth."

This is the signature item for the Ruth's Chris chain. It's a delicious filet mignon that comes to your table sizzling hot and does seem to melt in your mouth as the menu claims. If you want to prepare filets the Ruth's Chris way you first need some corn-fed filets, which can be found in specialty meat markets or through mail-order outlets such as Omaha Steaks. If you can't find corn-fed beef, you can still use this cooking method with filet purchased at your supermarket, but the meat will likely not be as tasty and tender.

I've designed this recipe to duplicate the petite filet on the Ruth's Chris menu, since the larger filet is around 14 ounces. That size can be difficult to obtain unless you cut your own. Ruth's Chris uses a special broiler which reaches temperatures as high as 1800 degrees F. It's likely you don't have such an oven, so you will have to use a conventional oven set on high broil, with the rack placed up near the top. You want to be sure the filet is about 5 to 6 inches away from the heat source, and if you have gas, be very careful to watch for flame-ups from spattering. If you begin to get flames, move the rack to a lower level so that you don't start a fire. Also, you need to have ceramic oven-safe plates to serve this meat properly sizzling. This recipe assumes that your broiler is located at the top of the oven. If not, you won't be able to use this technique until you get a new oven. Sorry.

4 **8-ounce filet mignon steaks**	**Pepper**
6 **tablespoons butter, softened**	2 **teaspoons chopped fresh**
Salt	**parsley**

1. Preheat the broiler.
2. Prepare the filets by drying them with a cloth or paper towel

261

and rubbing ½ tablespoon of butter per steak over the top and bottom. Salt and pepper the filet.

3. Make sure your broiler is on high and that it is good and hot. It should have preheated for *at least* 30 minutes. Put four oven-safe ceramic serving plates on the bottom rack in the oven when you start to preheat the broiler and through the entire cooking time. Move another rack up to the top so that when you put the filets in they will be about 5 to 6 inches from the heat. You will have to check the filets periodically to be sure they haven't flamed up. Cook the meat in a broiler pan, turning halfway through cooking time for the following length of time based on your preference:

COOKING CHART

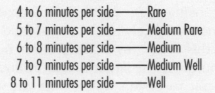

4. When the meat is done, carefully remove the ceramic plates from the oven. On each of them, place 1 tablespoon of butter. It should sizzle.
5. When the butter has melted, place a steak in the center of the plate.
6. Sprinkle a pinch of the parsley on top of the meat, and another pinch around it onto the butter.
7. Serve the dishes sizzling hot.

Tidbits

Try cooking other cuts of meat using this same method—delicious! Of course, the broiling time will vary depending on the thickness of your meat.

✳ Ruth's Chris Steak House Creamed Spinach

Serves 4 as a side dish

"Ruth's Chris Steak House" is such a difficult name to spit out that a restaurant critic suggested it be used as a sobriety test. Surely anyone who could say the name three times fast couldn't possibly be intoxicated. But the hard-to-say name has probably worked well for the steakhouse chain; it is surely a memorable one. The name came from the first restaurant that Ruth purchased in 1965 called Chris Steak House. When she opened a second restaurant with that same name, the previous owner, Chris Matu-lich, tried to sue her. She won the case, but to avoid future lawsuits she put her name in front of the original and it became the tongue twister we know today.

The delicious creamed spinach served at Ruth's Chris inspired this recipe that has just a hint of cayenne pepper in it for that Louisiana zing. The recipe requires a package of frozen spinach to make it convenient, but you can use the same amount of fresh spinach if you prefer.

1 10-ounce package frozen chopped spinach	½ cup heavy cream
2 tablespoons butter	¼ teaspoon salt
1½ tablespoons all-purpose flour	Dash pepper
	Dash nutmeg
	Dash cayenne pepper

1. Cook the spinach following the directions on the package. Drain and squeeze all the liquid from the spinach when it's done.
2. Melt the butter in a saucepan over medium heat. Be careful not to burn it.
3. Add the flour to the melted butter and stir until smooth.
4. Add the cream and heat for 2 to 3 minutes or until the sauce thickens. Stir constantly so that sauce does not burn.
5. Add the spinach, salt, pepper, nutmeg, and cayenne. Cook for 2 to 4 minutes, stirring often. Serve hot.

✳ Ruth's Chris Steak House Potatoes Au Gratin

Serves 4 to 6 as a side dish

Menu Description: *"In cream sauce, topped with melted sharp cheddar."*

There are many ways to order potatoes from the Ruth's Chris menu including steak fries, julienne fries, shoestring fries, cottage fries, Lyonnaise, baked, and au gratin.

Here is a traditional, classic recipe for the delicious side dish inspired by the Ruth's Chris creation. You may use less of the cream and milk mixture in your version depending on the size baking dish you use and the size of your potatoes. Stop adding the creamy mixture when it is level with the sliced potatoes in the baking dish. Be sure to use a casserole dish that has a lid for the first stage of the baking.

3 to 4 medium russet potatoes, peeled	¼ teaspoon salt
1 cup heavy cream	⅛ teaspoon pepper
½ cup milk	1 tablespoon butter, softened
1½ tablespoons flour	1½ cups grated Cheddar cheese
1 large clove garlic, pressed	1 teaspoon finely chopped fresh parsley

1. Preheat the oven to 400 degrees F.
2. Cut the potatoes into ¼-inch slices, then quarter each of those slices.
3. Beat together the cream, milk, flour, garlic, salt, and pepper by hand just until well combined.
4. Coat the inside of a large baking dish with the softened butter.
5. Arrange one-fourth of the potatoes on the bottom of the dish. Pour some of the cream mixture over the potatoes. Repeat this layering step three more times.
6. Cover the potatoes and bake for 20 minutes. Uncover, and bake another 40 minutes or until the potatoes are starting to brown on top.

7. Sprinkle grated cheese over the top of the potatoes and continue to bake for 5 to 10 minutes or until the cheese is melted and slightly browned and the potatoes are tender.
8. Sprinkle the parsley on top and serve.

✳ Shoney's Country Fried Steak

Serves 4 as an entree

Menu Description: "Tender steak, lightly breaded and golden fried. Smothered with country milk gravy."

Alex Schoenbaum opened the doors to his first restaurant, Parkette, a drive-in in Charleston, West Virginia, in 1947, at the start of a boom in popularity of the classic American drive-in restaurants many of us now know only from reruns of *Happy Days*. Schoenbaum's restaurant did very well and he decided, in 1951, to purchase a Big Boy franchise, the fastest growing chain at the time. In 1953, Parkette changed its name to Shoney's Big Boy.

Today Shoney's is no longer affiliated with Big Boy, but maintains a menu that features the Southern homestyle favorites that have made it so successful for so long. One of the old-time favorites is the Country Fried Steak smothered in peppered milk gravy. The technique here is to freeze the steaks after they have been breaded with flour. This way the coating won't wash off when the steaks are fried—the same technique the restaurants use.

2 cups all-purpose flour	2 cups water
2 teaspoons salt	4 4-ounce cube steaks
¼ teaspoon ground black pepper	Vegetable oil for frying

Country gravy

1½ tablespoons ground beef	¼ teaspoon coarsely ground black pepper
¼ cup all-purpose flour	¼ teaspoon salt
2 cups chicken stock	
2 cups whole milk	

1. Prepare the steaks at least several hours before you plan to serve this meal. First, sift the flour, salt, and pepper together into a large, shallow bowl. Pour the water into another shallow bowl.

266

2. Trim the steaks of any fat, then use your hand to press down firmly on each cube steak on a hard surface to flatten it out a bit. You don't want the steaks too thick.
3. Dredge each steak, one at a time, first in the water and then in the flour. Repeat this one more time so that each steak has been coated twice.
4. When all four steaks have been coated, place them on waxed paper and put them into the freezer for several hours until they are solid. This is the same technique used at the restaurant chain to ensure that the flour coating won't fall off when frying the steaks.
5. About 10 minutes before you are ready to cook the steaks, prepare the gravy by browning the ground beef in a small frying pan. Crumble the meat into tiny pieces as you cook it.
6. Transfer the meat to a medium saucepan over medium heat. Add ¼ cup flour and stir it in with the ground beef. Add the remaining ingredients for the gravy and bring to a boil, stirring often. Cook for 10 to 15 minutes until thick. Reduce the heat to low to keep the gravy warm while the steaks are prepared.
7. As the gravy is cooking, heat oil in a deep fryer or a deep frying pan over medium/high heat to 350 degrees F. You want enough oil to cover the steaks when frying.
8. When the oil is hot, drop the steaks, one at a time, into the oil. Fry for 8 to 10 minutes or until golden brown, then drain on paper towels.
9. Serve the steaks with gravy poured over the top, with a side of mashed potatoes, grits, or steamed vegetables, if desired.

* Shoney's
Slow-Cooked Pot Roast

Serves 6 to 8 as an entree

Menu Description: *"Tender roast beef and carrots slow-simmered and served in a rich brown gravy."*

Remember Mom's delicious pot roast? Shoney's tender slow-cooked entree is just as good, if not better than, many home recipes. The secret to making tender, flaky pot roast is the long slow-cooking process with frequent basting—and then cooking in the pan juices after flaking the meat. This recipe, based on Shoney's popular dish, requires 3 to 4 hours of cooking to make the meat tender. The meat is then flaked apart, put back into the pot with the pan juices and carrots, and cooked more to infuse the meat with flavor. The original recipe requires a rump roast, a tough cut of meat before cooking, which is reasonably low in fat. If you like, you can also use the more tender and less costly chuck roast. This cut of meat requires about an hour less time in the oven to tenderize it because of its higher fat content.

Pot roast

2 tablespoons butter	1½ teaspoons fresh thyme
1 4-pound rump roast	(or ½ teaspoon dried)
1 onion, chopped	1½ teaspoons fresh parsley
2 stalks celery, chopped	(or ½ teaspoon dried)
1 bay leaf	2 cups beef stock or canned
1 large clove garlic,	beef broth
chopped	1 teaspoon salt
20 whole peppercorns	2 large carrots, sliced

Gravy

2 cups beef stock or canned	⅓ cup all-purpose flour
beef broth	Salt and pepper to taste

268

On the Side

Mashed potatoes

1. Preheat the oven to 325 degrees F.
2. Melt the butter in a large oven-safe pot or Dutch oven and sear all sides of the roast in the melted butter for 2 to 3 minutes per side, or until all sides are browned.
3. Remove the meat from the pot to a plate. Add the onion, celery, bay leaf, garlic, peppercorns, thyme, and parsley to the pot that the meat was in and sauté over high heat for 5 minutes until the onion starts to brown.
4. Put the roast back in the pot with the vegetables. Add the beef stock and ½ teaspoon salt.
5. Cook the meat in the oven, covered, for 4 hours or until the meat is tender enough to tear apart. Every half hour or so baste the meat with the broth so that it doesn't dry out.
6. When the roast is tender, remove it from the pot and strain the stock into a medium bowl. Discard the vegetables and spices, but keep the stock.
7. Using two forks, shred the roast apart into slightly bigger than bite-size chunks. Put the meat back into the pot and pour the stock over it. Add the remaining ½ teaspoon salt and the carrots.
8. Put the pot back into the oven and cook for 40 to 50 minutes. This will make the meat even more tender and fill it with flavor. By this time the carrots should be tender.
9. Just before serving the pot roast make a gravy by straining the stock from the pot roast and combining it with an additional 2 cups of beef stock. Sprinkle the flour into a medium saucepan and stir in the liquid. (You should have about 3 cups of stock altogether. If not, add water until you have 3 cups of liquid.) Bring the mixture to a boil, stirring often until thick. Remove from the heat.
10. Serve the pot roast and carrots on a bed of mashed potatoes with the gravy poured over the top. Salt and pepper to taste.

✱ Shoney's
Hot Fudge Cake

Serves 12

Menu Description: *"Vanilla ice cream between two pieces of devil's food cake. Served with hot fudge, creamy topping and a cherry."*

One of Shoney's signature dessert items is this Hot Fudge Cake, a dessert worshipped by all who taste it. It's such a simple recipe for something that tastes so good. To make construction of this treat simpler for you, the recipe calls for a prepackaged devil's food cake mix like that which you can find in just about any supermarket baking aisle. Bear in mind when you shop for ingredients for this recipe that the vanilla ice cream must come in a box, so that the ice cream slices can be arranged properly between the cake layers. Leftovers can be frozen and served up to several weeks later.

1 18.25-ounce box devil's food cake mix	1 16-ounce jar chocolate fudge topping
3 eggs	1 can whipped cream
1⅓ cups water	12 maraschino cherries
⅓ cup vegetable oil	
1 half-gallon box vanilla ice cream (must be in a box)	

1. Mix the batter for the cake as instructed on the box of the cake mix by combining cake mix, eggs, water, and vegetable oil in a large mixing bowl.
2. Measure only 4 cups of the batter into a well-greased 12 × 8-inch baking pan. This will leave about 1 cup of batter in the bowl, which you can discard or use for another recipe, such as cupcakes.
3. Bake the cake according to the box instructions. Allow the cake to cool completely.
4. When the cake has cooled, carefully remove it from the pan,

and place it right side up onto a sheet of wax paper. With a long knife (a bread knife works great) slice horizontally through the middle of the cake, and carefully remove the top.

5. Pick up the wax paper with the bottom of the cake still on it, and place it back into the baking pan.

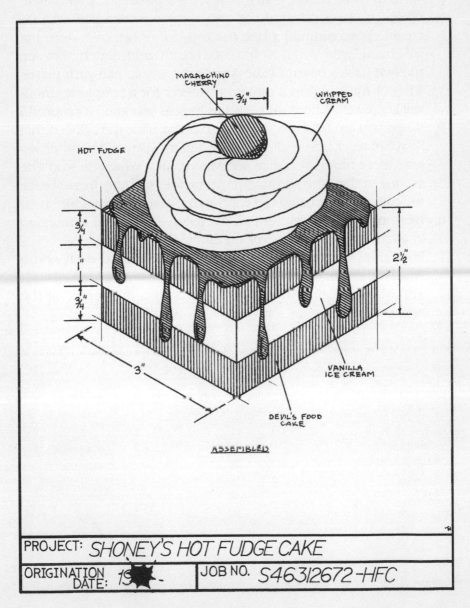

PROJECT: *SHONEY'S HOT FUDGE CAKE*

ORIGINATION DATE: 19 ██ -   JOB NO. *S46312672-HFC*

6. Take the ice cream from the freezer and, working quickly, tear the box open so that you can slice it like bread.
7. Make six ¾-inch-thick slices and arrange them on the cake bottom in the pan. Cover the entire surface of the cake with ice cream. You will most likely have to cut 2 of the ice cream slices in half to make it all fit. Hey, it's a puzzle . . . that melts!
8. When you have covered the entire bottom cake half with ice cream slices, carefully place the top half of the cake onto the ice cream layer. You now have ice cream sandwiched between the two halves of your cake. Cover the whole pan with plastic wrap or foil and pop it into your freezer for a couple hours (it will keep well in here for weeks as long as you keep it covered.)
9. When you are ready to serve the dessert, slice the cake so that it will make 12 even slices—slice lengthwise twice and cross-wise three times. You may not want to slice what you won't be serving at the time so that the remainder will stay fresh. Leave the cake you are using out for 5 minutes to defrost a bit.
10. Heat up the fudge either in a microwave or in a jar immersed in a saucepan of water over medium/low heat.
11. Pour the hot fudge over the cake slices and to each add a small mountain of whipped cream.
12. Top off each cake with a cherry stuck into the center of the whipped cream.

✳ Sizzler
Cheese Toast

Serves 2 to 4

In Los Angeles in 1957, Del Johnson noticed an article in the *Wall Street Journal* about a successful $1.09 per steak steakhouse chain with locations in New York, Chicago, and San Francisco. Inspired by the article, Del decided to open his own steakhouse in L.A., but with a twist that would save him money. His idea was to develop a steakhouse where customers would order their food at a food counter and pick it up when it was ready. Doesn't sound that exciting, but the concept was a hit. After the first Sizzler was open for a year, Del decided to run a two-day, one-cent anniversary sale: buy one steak at the regular price and get a second for just a penny. Del said, "We opened at 11:00. People were lined up from 11:00 until 9:00 at night, and we sold 1050 steaks in one day and about 1200 the second day."

With every meal, Sizzler serves a slice of tasty cheese toast. It's a simple recipe that goes well with just about any entree.

4 tablespoons butter	**4 teaspoons Kraft grated**
4 slices thick-sliced French	**Parmesan cheese**
bread	

1. Melt the butter in a small saucepan or in the microwave.
2. Use a brush to spread the butter evenly over one face of each slice of bread.
3. Sprinkle the Parmesan cheese over the butter.
4. Grill the bread, buttered side down, on a frying pan or griddle over medium/low heat for 5 minutes or until golden brown. Grill only the buttered side.

✳ Sizzler
Chicken Club Sandwich

Serves 1 as an entree (can be doubled)

When Del Johnson and his wife were trying to think of a name for their new restaurant concept they were looking for the perfect single-word name. "Something that would merchandise well," said Del. "In the old days, they served steaks on those sizzling platters. In a first class restaurant when you ordered a steak, they'd bring it out, put the butter on that steak and that plate was hot, it was aluminum and it would sizzle when they put it down in front of you. That's how we came up with the name. I knew we wanted to use those sizzling platters."

Eventually the restaurant would diversify the menu to include items other than the sizzling steak. One of those on the menu today is the chicken club sandwich, which you can now easily duplicate at home.

1 **boneless, skinless chicken breast half**	1 **slice Swiss cheese**
Vegetable oil	2 **slices bacon, cooked**
Salt	1 **small slice onion, separated**
1 **hamburger bun**	2 **slices tomato**
¼ **cup chopped lettuce**	½ **tablespoon Thousand Island dressing**

1. Prepare the barbecue or preheat the stovetop grill or broiler.
2. Lightly brush the chicken breast with oil, and grill it over medium heat for 5 minutes per side or until done. Salt the chicken.
3. Brown the faces of the bun top and bottom on the grill or in a skillet over medium heat.
4. Stack the sandwich in the following order from the bottom up:
   a. bottom bun
   b. lettuce
   c. chicken breast
   d. Swiss cheese

e. bacon slices, crisscrossed

f. onion

g. tomato slices

5. Spread the Thousand Island dressing on the face of the top bun, and top off your sandwich with it.

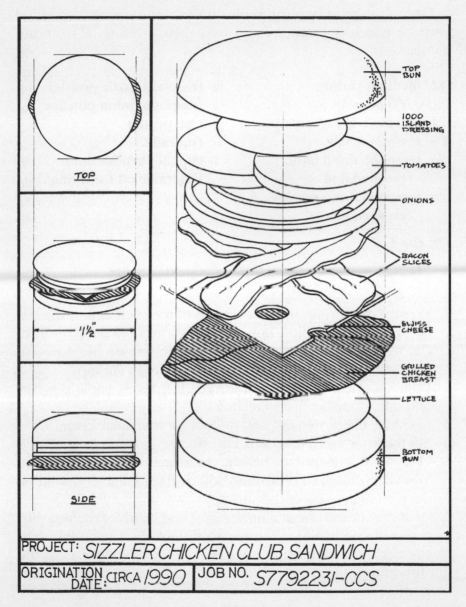

TOP

SIDE

1½"

TOP BUN

1000 ISLAND DRESSING

TOMATOES

ONIONS

BACON SLICES

SWISS CHEESE

GRILLED CHICKEN BREAST

LETTUCE

BOTTOM BUN

PROJECT: SIZZLER CHICKEN CLUB SANDWICH

ORIGINATION DATE: CIRCA 1990

JOB NO. S7792231-CCS

✳ Sizzler
Southern Fried Shrimp

Serves 1 as an entree, or 2 as an appetizer

One of the most popular items on the Sizzler menu is the fried shrimp, which is often offered as a belly-stuffing, all-you-can-eat deal.

12 medium shrimp (⅓ pound)	⅛ teaspoon garlic powder
1 cup plain bread crumbs	⅛ teaspoon onion powder
1½ teaspoons salt	1 egg, beaten
½ teaspoon dried basil, crushed fine	½ cup milk
½ teaspoon dried parsley, crushed fine	1 cup all-purpose flour
	Vegetable oil for frying

On the Side

Lemon wedge   Cocktail sauce

1. Prepare the shrimp by removing all of the shell except the last section and the tailfins. Butterfly the shrimp by cutting most of the way through along the back of the shrimp on the side with the dark vein. Remove the vein and rinse each shrimp.
2. Combine the bread crumbs, salt, basil, parsley, garlic powder, and onion powder in a small bowl.
3. Combine the beaten egg and milk in another small bowl.
4. Sift the flour into a third small bowl.
5. Heat oil in a deep fryer or large saucepan over medium heat. You want the oil to be around 350 degrees F and it should be deep enough to cover the shrimp.
6. Coat the shrimp one at a time, using one hand for the wet mixture and one hand for the dry stuff. First dip the shrimp into the egg and milk mixture, then drop it into the flour. Coat the shrimp with the flour with the dry hand and then drop it back

into the milk mixture. When it's completely moistened drop it into the bread crumbs and coat it again. Set each shrimp on a plate until all of them are coated.

7. Drop the shrimp into the hot oil and cook for 3 to 4 minutes or until the outside is golden. Serve with a wedge of lemon and cocktail sauce for dipping.

Tidbits

This is also great with cornflake crumbs rather than bread crumbs.

✳ Stuart Anderson's Black Angus Cheesy Garlic Bread

Serves 2 to 4

Recent years have brought a surge in steakhouse chains across the country. But before there was Lone Star, Outback, or Ruth's Chris, a real rancher named Stuart Anderson was serving up huge cuts of delicious prime beef in his Seattle-based restaurant chain. The first Black Angus restaurant opened on April Fool's Day in 1964 and quickly became known for its huge, juicy cuts of prime rib.

Early on, Stuart Anderson's Black Angus served a signature bread dubbed "Ranch Bread" free with each meal. Around five years ago that evolved into Cheesy Garlic Bread, which is no longer free, but is still a delicious and often requested side for any meal. Try to find a large loaf of French or Italian bread for this recipe. The recipe works with just about any type of bread loaf, but to make it more like the original, bigger is better.

1 tablespoon shredded Cheddar cheese	½ teaspoon minced green onion (the white part only)
2 tablespoons shredded Monterey Jack cheese	Dash salt
2 tablespoons grated Parmesan cheese	2 tablespoons butter
1 teaspoon chopped fresh parsley	½ clove garlic, pressed
	¼ loaf French or Italian bread (see Tidbits)

1. Preheat the oven to 450 degrees F.
2. Use finely shredded Cheddar and Monterey Jack cheese for this recipe. If you buy your cheese already shredded and it seems coarse, use a knife to chop it up a bit before you combine it with the other ingredients.
3. Add the Parmesan, parsley, onion, and salt to the cheese blend.
4. In a large frying pan or skillet, melt the butter over low heat.

278

5. Add the garlic to the butter. Be sure the heat is very low or the garlic could scorch and become bitter.
6. Slice a loaf of French bread in half, then cut one of the halves lengthwise through the middle.

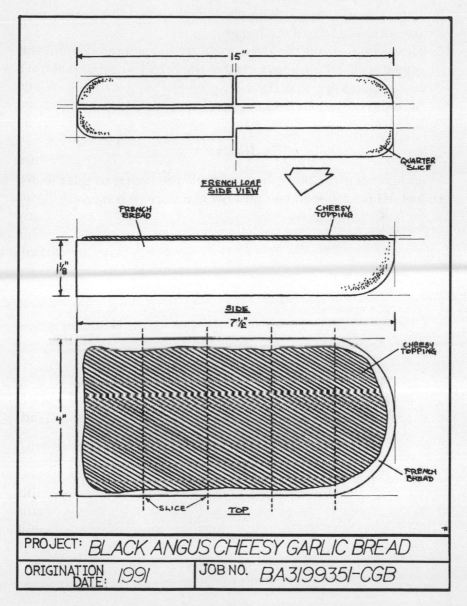

15"

QUARTER SLICE

FRENCH LOAF
SIDE VIEW

FRENCH BREAD

CHEESY TOPPING

1⅛"

SIDE
7½"

CHEESY TOPPING

4"

FRENCH BREAD

SLICE   TOP

PROJECT: BLACK ANGUS CHEESY GARLIC BREAD

ORIGINATION DATE: 1991

JOB NO. BA319935I-CGB

7. Take that quarter loaf of bread and invert it, face down, in the pan of butter. The bread will soak up some of the garlic butter. Be sure the entire face of the bread has been coated with butter.
8. Brush the crust of the bread with butter from the pan while it sits in the pan face down.
9. Put the bread on a baking sheet and spread the cheese mixture over the face of the bread.
10. Heat the bread in the oven for 8 to 10 minutes or until the edges begin to turn brown. Give the bread a quick broil for 1 to 2 minutes just to make it crispier.
11. Slice the bread into 5 equal pieces and serve hot.

Tidbits

You may want to double or quadruple the recipe to use the entire loaf of bread, depending on how many are to be served.

✳ Stuart Anderson's
Black Angus Western T-bone

Serves 2 as an entree

Menu Description: "A huge, savory, 16 oz. bone-in U.S.D.A. choice steak, prepared with a smoky marinade and fire-grilled. Smothered with sautéed mushrooms, roasted red peppers and real smoked bacon."

"Come in for dinner and I'll do the dishes," Stuart Anderson used to promise in television ads. Stuart had a down-home appeal that worked wonders for his chain. Stuart was a rancher who raised a small number of cattle, Clydesdales, and sheep for many years, and was known for his casual, laid-back approach to just about everything. When he opened the first restaurant he built it on a "ranch-to-restaurant" philosophy, meaning that he could supply the fresh beef from his own small ranch, or at least imply that was the case. But as the dinner house's popularity exploded over the years, larger suppliers had to be called upon to deliver the beef to the growing chain. Still, the fable lived on, and it worked very well for the restaurant. Even with more than one hundred stores in the chain, customers continued to believe they were getting home-grown steaks picked by old Stuart himself—a rumor that Stuart would neither confirm nor deny.

Now you can hand pick your own T-bone steaks when you whip up this recipe for steak in a smoky marinade that clones the Stuart Anderson's Black Angus recipe. The recipe here is for T-bone steaks, but you can use the marinade and topping on any cut of steak. If you can, plan on marinating the steaks overnight for the best flavor.

Smoky Marinade

4 teaspoons liquid smoke
2 teaspoons salt
1 clove garlic, pressed
  Dash ground black pepper

2 teaspoons vegetable oil
½ cup water
¼ teaspoon onion powder
¼ teaspoon minced fresh parsley

2 16-ounce T-bone steaks

281

Topping

2 tablespoons butter
2 cups sliced mushrooms
1 tablespoon diced roasted red pepper (canned is fine)
1 tablespoon diced sun-dried tomatoes (bottled in oil)

2 slices bacon, cooked and crumbled
Pinch chopped fresh parsley
Pinch dried thyme
Salt
½ teaspoon vinegar

1. Combine all of the ingredients for the smoky marinade in a medium bowl.
2. Pour the marinade over the T-bone steaks. You may want to use a large, sealable plastic bag for this. If you don't have one, be sure you use a covered container. Marinate the meat in your refrigerator for at least 4 hours. Overnight is best.
3. When you are ready to grill the steaks, preheat your barbecue.
4. As the barbecue heats, prepare the sautéed mushroom topping by melting the butter in a large skillet over medium heat.
5. Add the mushrooms, roasted peppers, and tomatoes to the butter. Sauté for about 5 minutes or until the mushrooms begin to turn brown on the edges.
6. Add the bacon, parsley, thyme, salt, and vinegar to the mushrooms and keep warm over low heat until the steaks are done.
7. When your grill is hot, cook the steaks for 3 to 5 minutes per side or until they are done to your liking. Salt the steaks to taste. Serve the steaks with the mushroom topping spooned over the top.

✳ Stuart Anderson's Black Angus Whiskey Pepper Steak

Serves 2 as an entree

Menu Description: *"U.S.D.A. choice top sirloin, fire grilled to your liking then doused with a whiskey pepper sauce."*

When the number of Black Angus restaurants had reached 117 by the early eighties, the Marriott Corporation stepped in to buy the chain from owner Stuart Anderson. Now, nearing 70, Stuart relaxes at his home on Whidby Island off the coast of Washington State, and spends his winters at his other home in warm Palm Springs, California.

Here is an easy recipe for sirloin pepper steak with a tasty whiskey sauce inspired by the popular dish served at Black Angus. Black Angus chefs probably got the idea for this dish from a classic French dish called *steak au poivre* in which the meat is covered with coarsely ground black pepper before being sautéed or broiled. Brandy or cognac is used to get the steak flaming for an elaborate presentation.

You won't have to set your steak on fire in this version. Though you will find that the flavorful sauce goes well with other cuts of steak besides the top sirloin called for here.

Whiskey Pepper Sauce

- 1 tablespoon butter
- 2 tablespoons chopped white onion
- 2 cups beef stock or canned beef broth
- ¼ teaspoon cracked black pepper
- 1 clove garlic, pressed
- 2 tablespoons whiskey
- 1 green onion, chopped
- 1 teaspoon cornstarch
- 1 tablespoon water

Pepper Steak

1 **16-ounce sirloin steak, cut**
   into two portions
2 **teaspoons cracked black**
   pepper

2 **tablespoons butter**
   Salt

1. Fire up the barbecue.
2. In a saucepan or deep skillet, make the whiskey pepper sauce by sautéing the white onions in the butter over high heat. In about 3 minutes the onions will begin to turn brown.
3. Add 1 cup of the beef stock to the onions. Add the cracked black pepper and garlic at this point as well. Continue to simmer over medium/high heat until the sauce has reduced by about half.
4. Add the whiskey, green onion, and remaining 1 cup of beef stock to the sauce and let it simmer over low heat while you prepare the steaks.
5. Spread ½ teaspoon of cracked pepper over the entire surface of each side of the sirloin steaks and press it into the steaks so that it sticks.
6. Melt 2 tablespoons of butter in a large skillet over medium/high heat. Drop the steaks into the melted butter and sear each side of the steaks for 1½ to 2 minutes or until brown.
7. When the barbecue is good and hot, grill the steaks for 3 to 5 minutes per side or until they are done to your liking. Salt the steaks lightly as they grill.
8. When the steaks are just about done, combine the cornstarch with the tablespoon of water in a small bowl. Stir just until the cornstarch dissolves.
9. Remove the whiskey sauce from the heat and add the cornstarch to it. Put the sauce back on the heat and continue to cook on low until the sauce is thickened to the consistency you desire. Serve the steak doused with whiskey pepper sauce.

✳ T.G.I. Friday's Potato Skins

Serves 2 to 4 as an appetizer or snack

Menu Description: "Loaded with cheddar cheese and bacon. Served with sour cream and chives."

Perfume salesman Alan Stillman was a single guy in New York City in 1965, looking for a way to meet women who lived in his neighborhood. He figured a hip way to get their attention: buy a broken-down beer joint in the area, jazz it up, and call it "The T.G.I.F." to attract the career crowd. Within a week, police had to barricade the area to control the crowds flocking to Alan's new restaurant. The restaurant made $1 million in its first year—a lot of dough back then. Soon restaurateurs were imitating the concept across the country.

In 1974 T.G.I. Friday's invented an appetizer that would also be imitated by many others in the following years. Today Potato Skins are still the most popular item on the T.G.I. Friday's menu, with nearly 4 million orders served every year. The recipe has the added benefit of providing you with leftover baked potato ready for mashing or to use in another dish.

4 **medium russet potatoes**	¼ **cup (½ stick) butter, melted**
⅓ **cup sour cream**	1½ **cups shredded Cheddar**
1 **tablespoon snipped fresh**	**cheese**
chives	5 **slices bacon, cooked**

1. Preheat the oven to 400 degrees F. Bake the potatoes for 1 hour. Let the potatoes cool down enough so that you can touch them.
2. As the potatoes are baking, make the sour cream dip by mixing the sour cream with the chives. Place the mixture in a covered container in your refrigerator.
3. When the potatoes are cool enough to handle, make 2 lengthwise cuts through each potato, resulting in three ½- to ¾-inch

slices. Discard the middle slices or save them for a separate dish of mashed potatoes. This will leave you with two potato skins per potato.

4. With a spoon, scoop some of the potato out of each skin, being sure to leave about ¼ inch of potato inside of the skin.

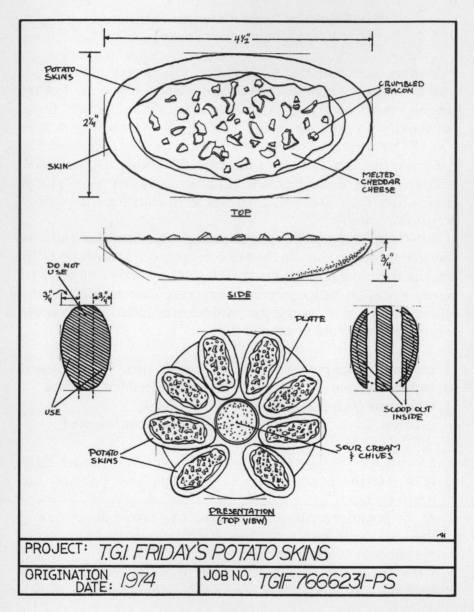

PROJECT: *T.G.I. FRIDAY'S POTATO SKINS*

ORIGINATION DATE: *1974*

JOB NO. *TGIF 7666231-PS*

5. Brush the entire surface of each potato skin, inside and outside, with the melted butter.
6. Place the skins on a cookie sheet, cut side up, and broil them for 6 to 8 minutes or until the edges begin to turn dark brown.
7. Sprinkle 2 to 3 tablespoons of Cheddar cheese into each skin.
8. Crumble the cooked bacon and sprinkle 1 to 2 teaspoons of the bacon pieces onto the cheese.
9. Broil the skins for 2 more minutes or until the cheese is thoroughly melted. Serve hot, arranged on a plate surrounding a small bowl of the sour cream dip.

✳ T.G.I. Friday's Nine-Layer Dip

Serves 4 to 8 as an appetizer or snack

Menu Description: "Refried Beans, cheddar cheese, guacamole,
black olives, seasoned sour cream, green onions, tomatoes and cilantro.
Served with tortilla chips and fresh salsa."

When the first T.G.I. Friday's opened in New York City in 1965 as a meeting place for single adults, *Newsweek* and *The Saturday Evening Post* reported that it was the beginning of the "singles age." Today the restaurant's customers have matured, many are married, and they bring their children with them to the more than 300 Friday's across the country and around the world.

The Nine-Layer Dip is one of the often requested appetizers on the T.G.I. Friday's menu. This dish will serve half a dozen people easily, so it's perfect for a small gathering, or as a snack. Don't worry if there's only a couple of you—leftovers can be refrigerated for a day or two. Cilantro, also called fresh coriander or Chinese parsley, can be found in the produce section of most supermarkets near the parsley.

⅔ cup sour cream
⅛ teaspoon cumin
⅛ teaspoon cayenne pepper
⅛ teaspoon paprika
  Dash salt
1 16-ounce can refried beans
1 cup shredded Cheddar cheese

½ cup guacamole (made fresh or frozen, thawed)
¼ cup sliced black olives
2 green onions, chopped (¼ cup)
1 medium tomato, chopped
1 teaspoon chopped fresh cilantro

On the Side

Salsa

1. Combine the sour cream, cumin, cayenne pepper, paprika, and salt in a small bowl and mix well. Set aside.

288

2. Heat the refried beans until hot, using a microwave or in a saucepan over medium heat.
3. When the beans are hot, spread them over the center of a serving platter or in a shallow dish.
4. Sprinkle ½ of the cheese evenly over the beans.
5. Spread the guacamole over the cheese.

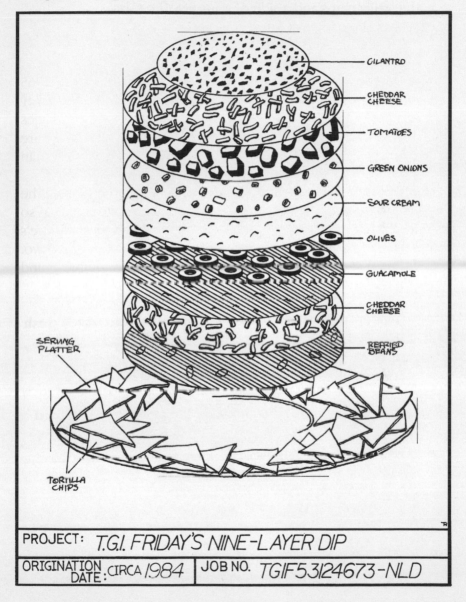

CILANTRO

CHEDDAR CHEESE

TOMATOES

GREEN ONIONS

SOUR CREAM

OLIVES

GUACAMOLE

CHEDDAR CHEESE

REFRIED BEANS

SERVING PLATTER

TORTILLA CHIPS

PROJECT: *T.G.I. FRIDAY'S NINE-LAYER DIP*

ORIGINATION DATE: CIRCA *1984*   JOB NO. *TGIF53124673-NLD*

6. Sprinkle the sliced olives over the guacamole.
7. Spread the seasoned sour cream over the olives.
8. Sprinkle the green onions, then the tomatoes evenly over the sour cream layer.
9. Finish up by sprinkling the remainder of the cheese over the tomatoes, and topping the dip off with the cilantro. Serve the dip with tortilla chips and a side of your favorite salsa.

✳ T.G.I. Friday's California Chargrilled Turkey Sandwich

Serves 4 as an entree

Menu Description: "Chargrilled all-white meat turkey burger, served on a toasted whole wheat bun with lettuce, tomatoes, alfalfa sprouts, onions and avocado."

Noting the success of the first T.G.I. Friday's in New York City, a group of fun-loving Dallas businessmen opened the first franchise store. The investors decorated their Dallas T.G.I. Friday's with fun antiques and collectibles gathered from around the countryside—and now all of the Friday's are decorated that way. Six months after the opening of the Dallas location, waiters and waitresses began doing skits and riding bicycles and roller skates around the restaurant. That's also when the now defunct tradition of ringing in every Friday evolved. Thursday night at midnight was like a New Year's Eve party at T.G.I. Friday's, with champagne, confetti, noisemakers, and a guy jumping around in a gorilla suit as if he had a few too many espressos.

Here's a favorite of burger lovers who don't care where the beef is. It's an alternative to America's most popular food with turkey instead of beef, plus some alfalfa sprouts and avocado to give it a "California" twist.

Honey Mustard Sauce

¼ cup mayonnaise	1 tablespoon honey
1 tablespoon yellow mustard (like French's)	½ teaspoon sesame oil
	½ teaspoon distilled vinegar

1 pound ground turkey (all-white meat if available)	4 romaine lettuce leaves
Salt	½ cup alfalfa sprouts (a handful)
Pepper	1 medium tomato, sliced
4 whole wheat hamburger buns	1 to 2 slices white onion
Soft butter	1 ripe avocado, sliced

291

1. Prepare the barbecue or preheat the stovetop grill.
2. Combine the mayonnaise, mustard, honey, oil, and vinegar in a small bowl. Cover and keep refrigerated until later.
3. Divide the ground turkey into four even portions and on wax paper pat out four ½-inch-thick patties with the same diameter as the buns.

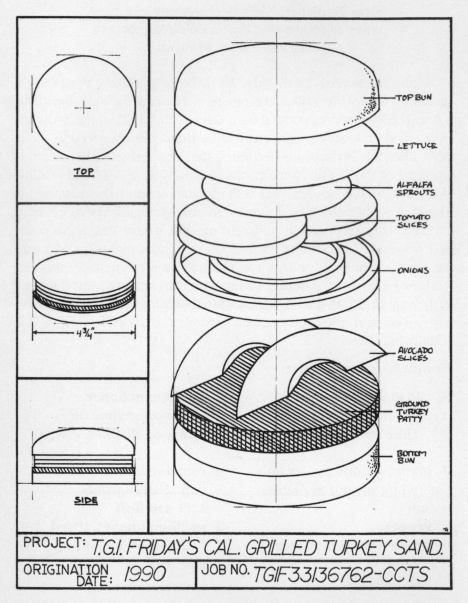

TOP

4¾"

SIDE

TOP BUN

LETTUCE

ALFALFA SPROUTS

TOMATO SLICES

ONIONS

AVOCADO SLICES

GROUND TURKEY PATTY

BOTTOM BUN

PROJECT: *T.G.I. FRIDAY'S CAL. GRILLED TURKEY SAND.*

ORIGINATION DATE: *1990*   JOB NO. *TGIF33I36762-CCTS*

4. Grill these patties for 6 to 8 minutes per side or until done. Be sure to salt and pepper both sides of each patty.
5. Prepare the buns by lightly buttering the face of the tops and bottoms, and then grilling them in a hot skillet until brown.
6. The sandwich is served "open face" so that the customer can put the hot side and the cold side together at the table (remember the McD.L.T?). Build the cold side of the sandwich by inverting the top bun and stacking the ingredients on it in the following order from the bottom up:
   a. top bun (face up)
   b. lettuce leaf
   c. alfalfa sprouts
   d. 1 to 2 tomato slices
   e. 2 onion rings (from the separated slices)
   f. 2 avocado slices
7. Arrange the bottom bun on the same plate. Add the hot ground turkey patty on the face of the bun and serve with the honey mustard dressing on the side.

Tidbits

Some tasty variations of this sandwich include adding slices of cooked bacon, or substituting barbecue sauce for the honey mustard.

* T.G.I. Friday's
Spicy Cajun Chicken Pasta

Serves 2 as a large entree

Menu Description: "Fettuccine tossed with sautéed chicken, mushrooms, onions and red and green peppers in Friday's own spicy, tomato Creole sauce."

There are over 360 T.G.I. Friday's restaurants in 44 states and 22 countries, all serving this Cajun-style chicken pasta. This dish is a bit like a jambalaya except the rice has been replaced with pasta.

Use a large pan for this recipe, and note that for the chicken stock or broth, you can also use a chicken bouillon cube dissolved in boiling water.

This recipe makes two large restaurant-size portions, but could easily serve a family of four.

4 **tablespoons (½ stick) butter**	1 **cup chicken stock** *or*
1 **green bell pepper, chopped**	1 **chicken bouillon cube**
(1 cup)	**dissolved in 1 cup boiling**
1 **red bell pepper, chopped**	**water**
(1 cup)	**Salt**
½ **white onion, sliced and**	¼ **teaspoon cayenne pepper**
quartered (1 cup)	¼ **teaspoon paprika**
1 **clove garlic, pressed**	¼ **teaspoon white pepper**
2 **boneless, skinless chicken**	¼ **teaspoon dried thyme**
breast halves	4 **to 6 quarts water**
2 **teaspoons olive oil**	1 **12-ounce box fettuccine**
1 **medium tomato, chopped**	2 **teaspoons chopped fresh**
4 **to 6 mushrooms, sliced**	**parsley**
(1¼ cup)	

1. Melt 2 tablespoons of the butter in a large skillet over medium/high heat.
2. Sauté the bell peppers, onions, and garlic in the butter for 8 to 10 minutes or until the vegetables begin to soften slightly.

3. As the vegetables are cooking, cut the chicken breasts into bite-size pieces.
4. Prepare a medium-size pan over high heat with the olive oil. When the pan is hot, add the chicken and cook, stirring, for 5 to 7 minutes or until the chicken shows no pink.
5. When the vegetables are soft (about 10 minutes) add the chicken to the pan.
6. Add the tomatoes, mushrooms, chicken stock, ¼ teaspoon salt, cayenne pepper, paprika, white pepper, and thyme and continue to simmer for 10 to 12 minutes until it thickens.
7. In the meantime bring the water to a boil in a large pot. If you like, add a half tablespoon of salt to the water. Cook the fettuccine in the boiling water until done. This will take 10 to 12 minutes.
8. When the noodles are done, drain them and add the remaining 2 tablespoons of butter. The butter should melt quickly on the hot noodles. Toss the noodles to mix in the butter.
9. Serve the dish by dividing the noodles in half onto two plates. Divide the chicken and vegetable sauce evenly and spread it over the top of the noodles on each plate. Divide the parsley and sprinkle it over each serving.

Tidbits

If you want a thicker sauce, combine ½ teaspoon arrowroot or cornstarch with 2 tablespoons of white wine in a small bowl and stir to dissolve. Remove the pan from the heat before adding this thickener, stir it in, then put it back on the heat.

✱ T.G.I. Friday's
Friday's Smoothies

Each recipe serves 2

Menu Description: "Healthful, nonalcoholic frozen fruit drinks."
"Gold Medalist: Coconut and pineapple, blended with grenadine,
strawberries and bananas."
"Tropical Runner: Fresh banana, pineapple and
pina colada mix frozen with crushed ice."

From the "obscure statistics" file, T.G.I. Friday's promotional material claims the restaurant was the first chain to offer stone-ground whole wheat bread as an option to its guests. It was also the first chain to put avocados, bean sprouts, and Mexican appetizers on its menu.

Also a first: Friday's Smoothies. In response to growing demand for nonalcoholic drinks, T.G.I. Friday's created smoothies, a fruit drink now found on many other restaurants' menus. Here are recipes to clone two of the nine fruit blend varieties. Great on a sizzling afternoon.

Gold Medalist

8 ounces frozen strawberries
    (not in syrup—do not
    defrost)
1 banana
1 cup pineapple juice

2 tablespoons coconut cream
¼ cup grenadine
1 cup ice
2 fresh strawberries
    (for garnish)

1. Pour all of the ingredients except the 2 fresh strawberries in the order listed into a blender and blend on high speed for 15 to 30 seconds or until all the ice is crushed and the drink is smooth.
2. Garnish each drink with a fresh strawberry.

Tropical Runner

1 banana
1 8-ounce can crushed
    pineapple with juice

½ cup liquid pina colada mix
½ cup orange sherbet
2 cups ice

1. Cut the banana in half and slice two ¼-inch slices from the middle of the banana and set the two slices aside for garnish.
2. Put the rest of banana and the remaining ingredients into a blender in the order listed. Blend on high speed for 15 to 30 seconds, or until the drink is smooth and creamy.
3. Add 1 banana slice to the top of each drink as a garnish.

Tidbits

You've probably already thought of this, but these drinks make tasty cocktails too. Just add a little rum or vodka, and about ½ cup more ice, before blending.

✳ Tony Roma's World Famous Ribs

Serves 2 to 4 as an entree

Tony Roma had already been in the restaurant business for many years when he opened Tony Roma's Place in North Miami, Florida, in 1972. This casual diner featured food at reasonable prices, nightly live entertainment and the house specialty—baby back ribs. Soon, customers were traveling from miles away to get a taste of the succulent, mouth-watering ribs. One rib-lover came from Texas in 1976: Clint Murchison, Jr., a Texas financier and owner of the Dallas Cowboys. After sampling the baby backs, and claiming they were the best he'd ever tasted, he struck up a deal with Tony to purchase the majority of the U.S. rights to the company and planned for a major expansion. Today that plan has been realized with nearly 150 Tony Roma's restaurants in the chain pulling in over $250 million per year.

The famous barbecue ribs served at the restaurant have been judged the best in America at a national rib cook-off and have won more than 30 awards at other state and local competitions. The secret to the tender, melt-in-your-mouth quality of the ribs at Tony Roma's is the long, slow-cooking process. Here is the *Top Secret Recipes* version of the cooking technique followed by three varieties of the famous barbecue sauce. Note that the restaurant uses pork baby back ribs for the Original Baby Backs recipe, and pork spare ribs for the Carolina Honeys and Red Hots. Of course *you* can use these sauces interchangeably on the ribs *you* like best, including beef ribs.

The Technique

4 **pounds baby back pork ribs** *or*	**Barbecue sauce for coating (See recipes on following pages)**
4 **pounds pork spareribs**	

1. Often when you buy ribs at the butcher counter, you get a full rack of ribs that wouldn't fit on a plate. Usually you just have to cut these long racks in half to get the perfect serving size

298

(about 4 to 6 rib bones per rack). You'll likely have 4 of these smaller racks at about a pound each.

2. Preheat the oven to 300 degrees F.
3. Tear off 4 pieces of aluminum foil that are roughly 6 inches longer than the ribs.
4. Coat the ribs, front and back, with your choice of barbecue sauce. Place a rack of ribs, one at a time, onto a piece of foil lengthwise and wrap it tightly.
5. Place the ribs into the oven with the seam of the foil wrap facing up. Cook for 2 to 2½ hours, or until you see the meat of the ribs shrinking back from the cut ends of the bones by about ½ inch. This long cooking time will ensure that the meat will be very tender and fall off the bone.
6. Toward the end of the cooking time, prepare the barbecue.
7. Remove the ribs from the foil and smother them with additional barbecue sauce. Be sure to save some sauce for later.
8. Grill the ribs on the hot barbecue for 2 to 4 minutes per side, or just until you see several spots of charred blackened sauce. Watch for flames and do not burn!
9. When the ribs are done, use a sharp knife to slice the meat between each bone about halfway down. This will make it easier to tear the ribs apart when they are served.

   Serve the ribs piping hot with additional sauce on the side, if desired.

Tidbits

If you've got time to marinate these ribs in advance, do it. I've found these ribs are extraordinary when they've been soaking in barbecue sauce for 24 hours before cooking. Just prepare the ribs in the foil as described in the recipe and keep them in your fridge. Toss them, foil and all, into the oven the next day, 2 to 2½ hours before you plan to scarf out.

✳ Tony Roma's
Original Baby Backs

Serves 2 to 4 as an entree

Menu Description: "Our house specialty and award-winning ribs. Lean, tender, meaty pork ribs cut from the choicest tenderloin and basted with our original barbecue sauce. So tender the meat practically falls off the bone."

This is the sauce that made the chain famous. This version of the sauce uses a ketchup base, vinegar, dark corn syrup, and a bit of Tabasco for a slight zing. The chain uses their sauce on baby back ribs and has started selling it by the bottle in each restaurant. Now you can make a version of your own that is less costly than the bottled brand, and can be used on any cut of ribs, or even chicken.

Barbecue Sauce

1 cup ketchup	¼ teaspoon garlic powder
1 cup vinegar	¼ teaspoon onion powder
½ cup dark corn syrup	¼ teaspoon Tabasco pepper
2 teaspoons sugar	sauce
½ teaspoon salt	

4 pounds baby back pork ribs

1. Combine all of the ingredients for the barbecue sauce in a saucepan over high heat. Use a whisk to blend the ingredients until smooth.
2. When the mixture comes to a boil, reduce the heat and simmer uncovered.
3. In 30 to 45 minutes, when the mixture thickens, remove it from the heat. If you want a thicker sauce, heat it longer. If you make the sauce too thick, thin it with more vinegar.
4. Use baby back ribs and the cooking technique from page 299 to complete the recipe.

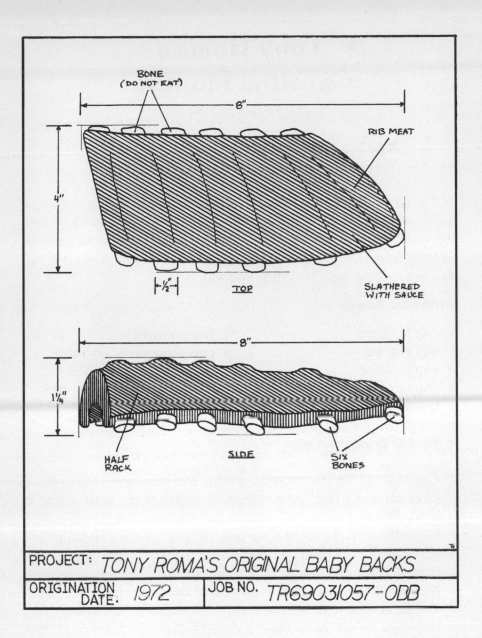

BONE
(DO NOT EAT)

8"

RIB MEAT

4"

1/2"

TOP

SLATHERED
WITH SAUCE

8"

1¼"

HALF
RACK

SIDE

SIX
BONES

PROJECT: *TONY ROMA'S ORIGINAL BABY BACKS*

ORIGINATION DATE: *1972*

JOB NO. *TR69031057-OBB*

✳ Tony Roma's Carolina Honeys

Serve 2 to 4 as an entree

Menu Description: "Tender select-cut pork spare ribs basted with our special-recipe sauce. Nothing could be finer . . ."

This smoky sauce is perfectly sweetened with honey and molasses, and bites just a bit with pepper sauce. Smother pork spareribs with this sauce, as they do at the restaurant chain. Also use it on baby back ribs and beef spare ribs along with the slow-cooking technique. It's good with chicken, too.

Barbecue Sauce

1 cup ketchup	½ teaspoon salt
1 cup vinegar	¼ teaspoon garlic powder
½ cup molasses	¼ teaspoon onion powder
½ cup honey	¼ teaspoon Tabasco pepper
1 teaspoon liquid smoke	sauce

4 pounds pork spare ribs

1. Combine all of the ingredients for the barbecue sauce in a saucepan over high heat. Blend the ingredients with a whisk until smooth.
2. When the mixture comes to a boil, reduce the heat and simmer uncovered.
3. In 30 to 45 minutes, when the mixture thickens, remove it from the heat. If you overcook it and make the sauce too thick, thin it with more vinegar.
4. Use pork spareribs and the cooking technique from page 299 to complete the recipe.

✳ Tony Roma's Red Hots

Serves 2 to 4 as an entree

Menu Description: "Some like it hot! Tender, meaty ribs basted with our spicy red hot sauce made with five types of peppers."

If you like your sauces especially spicy, this is the recipe for you. Five different peppers go into this one, including crushed red pepper, red bell pepper, Tabasco, cayenne pepper, and ground black pepper. The restaurant serves this one on pork spareribs, but you can slather it on any type of ribs, chicken, and steaks.

Barbecue Sauce

1 cup ketchup	½ teaspoon crushed red pepper flakes
1 cup vinegar	
½ cup dark corn syrup	½ teaspoon Tabasco pepper sauce
2 tablespoons molasses	
½ tablespoon finely diced red bell pepper	¼ teaspoon cayenne pepper
	¼ teaspoon ground black pepper
2 teaspoons sugar	
1 teaspoon liquid smoke	¼ teaspoon garlic powder
½ teaspoon salt	¼ teaspoon onion powder

4 pounds pork spareribs

1. Combine all of the ingredients for the barbecue sauce in a saucepan over high heat. Use a whisk to blend the ingredients until smooth.
2. When the mixture comes to a boil, reduce the heat and simmer uncovered.
3. In 30 to 45 minutes, when the mixture thickens, remove it from the heat. If you want a thicker sauce, cook it longer. If you make the sauce too thick, thin it with more vinegar.
4. Use pork spareribs and the cooking technique from page 299 to complete the recipe.

✳ Western Sizzlin "Teriyaki" Chicken Breast

Serves 2 as an entree

Western Sizzlin is a steakhouse similar in some ways to Sizzler, but the companies are not related. Although Western Sizzlin is known for its steak, the restaurant has a nice teriyaki chicken dish that is served topped with a slice of pineapple. You'll like this recipe since it includes a great way to make a delicious teriyaki sauce that you can use as a tasty marinade for a variety of dishes. It keeps well for weeks in the fridge. For the pineapple juice in the teriyaki recipe, you don't have to buy a separate can of juice. Instead you can use the juice that comes packed in the 5½-ounce can of pineapple slices that you use as garnish on the chicken—it's just the right amount for this recipe!

Teriyaki Sauce

¾ cup water	2 cloves garlic, quartered
½ cup soy sauce	⅓ cup sugar
1 slice onion, quartered (¼ inch thick)	⅓ cup pineapple juice (from canned pineapple slices)
2 nickel-size slices peeled gingerroot, halved	2 tablespoons vinegar
	1 tablespoon cornstarch

4 boneless, skinless chicken breast halves	4 canned pineapple slices in juice (5.5 ounce can)

1. Combine ½ cup water with the soy sauce in a small saucepan over high heat. Add the onion, gingerroot, and garlic. Bring the mixture to a boil, then reduce the heat and simmer for 10 minutes.
2. Strain off the onion, ginger, and garlic and return the liquid to the saucepan over low heat. Discard the vegetables.
3. Add the sugar, pineapple juice, and vinegar to the pan.
4. Combine the cornstarch with the remaining ¼ cup water in a small bowl and stir to dissolve any lumps. Remove the teriyaki mixture from the heat, add the cornstarch, then put it back on the

heat. Continue to simmer, stirring often, for 1 minute or so, until the mixture thickens. This will make about 1 cup of marinade.

5. When the teriyaki sauce has cooled, pour half of it over the chicken breasts arranged in a covered container or casserole dish. Keep the other half of the sauce for later to brush over the

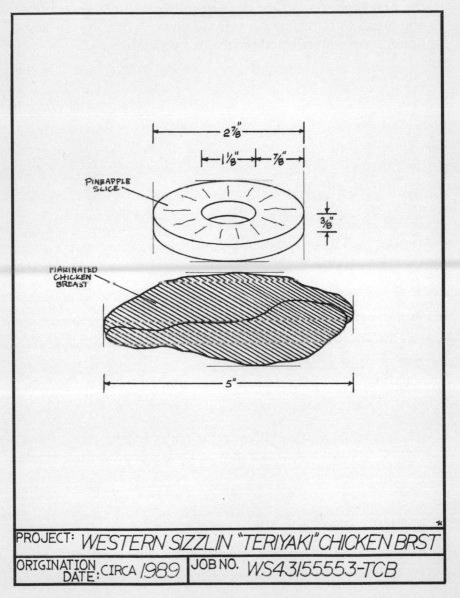

PROJECT: *WESTERN SIZZLIN "TERIYAKI" CHICKEN BRST*

ORIGINATION DATE: CIRCA *1989* JOB NO. *WS43155553-TCB*

chicken while it grills, and to serve on the side as additional marinade. Marinate the breasts in your refrigerator for at least 2 hours.

6. When you are ready to cook the chicken, preheat your barbecue or stovetop grill to high. Grill the chicken on each side for 5 to 7 minutes or until done. When you flip the chicken over the first time, put a slice of pineapple on top of each breast, and brush with the leftover teriyaki sauce. When the chicken is done, serve with rice and/or steamed vegetables.

BIBLIOGRAPHY

✳ ✳ ✳

Anderson, Henry W. *The Modern Foodservice Industry*. Dubuque, Iowa: William C. Brown Company Publishers, 1976.

Compton's New Media. *Compton's Interactive Encyclopedia*. Compton's New Media, Inc., 1992.

Grolier, Inc. *Grolier Multimedia Encyclopedia*. Danbury, CT: Grolier Electronic Publishing, Inc., 1995.

Herbst, Sharon Tyler. *Food Lover's Companion*. Hauppauge, New York: Barron's Educational Series, Inc., 1990.

Levenstein, Harvey. *Paradox of Plenty* New York: Oxford University Press, 1993.

Tennyson, Jeffrey. *Hamburger Heaven*. New York: Hyperion, 1992.

Ware, Richard, and James Rudnick. *The Restaurant Book*. New York: Facts on File Publications, 1986.

Witzel, Michael Karl. *The American Drive-In*. Osceola, WI: Motorbooks International Publishers and Wholesalers, 1994.

World Book, Inc. *The World Book Encyclopedia*. Chicago: World Book, Inc., 1986.

TRADEMARKS

* * *

Applebee's, Pizza Sticks, Club House Grille, and Tijuana "Philly" Steak Sandwich are registered trademarks of Applebee's International, Inc.

Benihana is a registered trademark of Benihana Inc.

Benningan's and Cookie Mountain Sundae are registered trademarks of Metromedia Co.

Big Boy is a registered trademark of Elias Brothers Restaurants, Inc.

California Pizza Kitchen is a registered trademark of California Pizza Kitchen, Inc.

Cap'n Crunch is a registered trademark of The Quaker Oats Company

The Cheesecake Factory is a registered trademark of The Cheesecake Factory, Inc.

Chi-Chi's and Mexican "Fried" Ice Cream are registered trademarks of Family Restaurants, Inc.

Chili's is a registered trademark of Brinker International

Cracker Barrel Old Country Store is a registered trademark of Cracker Barrel Old Country Store, Inc.

Denny's, Scram Slam, Moons Over My Hammy, and Super Bird are registered trademarks of Flagstar, Cos. Inc.

Dive!, Carrot Chips, Sicilian Sub Rosa, Brick Oven Mushroom and Turkey Cheese Sub, and Dive! S'mores are registered trademarks of Levy Restaurants, Inc.

Hard Rock Cafe and Famous Baby Rock Watermelon Ribs are registered trademarks of Hard Rock America, Inc., and Rank Organisation PLC

309

Hooters is a registered trademark of Hooters of America

Houlihan's, Houli Fruit Fizz, 'Shrooms, and Smashed Potatoes are registered trademarks of Houlihan's Restaurant Group, Inc.

IHOP and International House of Pancakes are registered trademarks of International House of Pancakes, Inc.

Lone Star Steakhouse & Saloon and Amarillo Cheese Fries are registered trademarks of Lone Star Steakhouse & Saloon, Inc.

Marie Callender's is a registered trademark of Marie Callender's Pie Shops, Inc.

The Olive Garden is a registered trademark of Darden Restaurants, Inc.

Outback Steakhouse, Bloomin' Onion, Walkabout Soup, and Alice Springs Chicken are registered trademarks of Outback Steakhouse, Inc.

Perkins and Granny's Country Omelette are registered trademarks of The Restaurant Co.

Pizza Hut is a registered trademark, and Stuffed Crust Pizza and Triple Decker Pizza are trademarks of Pizza Hut, Inc.

Planet Hollywood and Chicken Crunch are registered trademarks of Planet Hollywood (Region IV), Inc., in the United States and Canada, and Planet Hollywood International, Inc., elsewhere.

Poppers is a registered trademark of Anchor Foods, Inc.

Red Lobster is a registered trademark of Darden Restaurants, Inc.

Red Robin Burger & Spirits Emporium, No-Fire Peppers, and Mountain High Mudd Pie are registered trademarks of Skylark Co. Ltd.

Ruby Tuesday and Strawberry Tallcake are registered trademarks of Morrison Restaurants, Inc.

Ruth's Chris Steak House is a registered trademark of Ruth's Chris Steak House, Inc.

Shoney's is a registered trademark of Shoney's, Inc.

Sizzler is a registered trademark of Sizzler International, Inc.

Stuart Anderson's Black Angus is a registered trademark of American Restaurant Group, Inc.

T.G.I. Friday's and Friday's Smoothies are registered trademarks of T.G.I. Friday's, Inc.

Tony Roma's A Place for Ribs, Carolina Honeys, and Red Hots are registered trademarks of NPC International, Inc.

Western Sizzlin is a registered trademark of Western Sizzlin Corp.

INDEX

* * *

312

314

317

318